THE
ESTHETICIAN'S
GUIDE TO WORKING WITH
PHYSICIANS

THE ESTHETICIAN'S
GUIDE TO WORKING WITH
PHYSICIANS

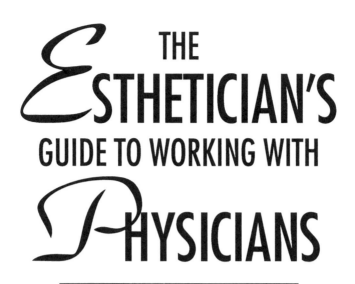

BY

SUSANNE S. WARFIELD

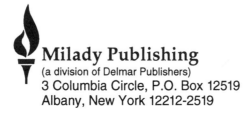

Milady Publishing
(a division of Delmar Publishers)
3 Columbia Circle, P.O. Box 12519
Albany, New York 12212-2519

NOTICE TO THE READER

Publisher and author do not warrant or guarantee any of the products described herein or perform any independent analysis in connection with any of the product information contained herein. Publisher and author do not assume, and expressly disclaim, any obligation to obtain and include information other than that provided to them by the manufacturer.

The reader is expressly warned to consider and adopt all safety precautions that might be indicated by the activities herein and to avoid all potential hazards. By following the instructions contained herein, the reader willingly assumes all risks in connections with such instructions.

The publisher and author make no representation or warranty of any kind, including but not limited to, the warranties of fitness for particular purpose or merchantability, nor are any such representations implied with respect to the material set forth herein, and the publisher and author take no responsibility with respect to such material. The publisher and author shall not be liable for any special, consequential, or exemplary damages resulting, in whole or part, from the readers' use of, or reliance upon, this material.

Cover Design: Suzanne Nelson
Cover Photo: Michael Dzaman Photography

Milady Staff
Publisher: Gordon Miller
Acquisitions Editor: Marlene McHugh Pratt
Project Editors: NancyJean Downey and Annette Downs Danaher
Production Manager: Brian Yacur
Production and Art/Design Coordinator: Suzanne Nelson

COPYRIGHT © 1997
Milady Publishing   and   Paramedical
(a division of Delmar Publishers)   Consultants, Inc.
an International Thomson Publishing company I⒯P®

Printed in the United States of America
Printed and distributed simultaneously in Canada

For more information, contact:
SalonOvations
Milady Publishing
3 Columbia Circle , Box 12519
Albany, New York   12212-2519

1 2 3 4 5 6 7 8 9 10   XXX   01 00 99 98 97 96

Library of Congress Cataloging-in-Publication Data

Warfield, Susanne S.
     SalonOvations' the esthetician's guide to working with physicians / by Susanne S. Warfield.
          p.   cm.
     Includes index.
     ISBN: 1-56253-311-8
     1. Medical rehabilitation.   2. Cosmetics.   3. Beauty operators.   4. Surgery, Plastic.
     5. Dermatology.   I. Title.
     [DNLM: 1. Allied Health Occupations. 2. Esthetics. 3. Vocational Guidance. W 21.5 W274s 1996]
RM930.W37 1996
617.9'5—dc20
DNLM/DLC   96-23284
for Library of Congress   CIP

Dedication

This book is dedicated to Ted and Barbara Schwenker, who have always supported me through the trials and tribulations of my life. You both believed and trusted in me and gave me the support I needed to make it through the tough times. Thanks, Mom and Dad!

From the Author

Cosmetic services have become one of the fastest growing segments of medical practice today. This fast growth inspired me to write this book, as a comprehensive guide to assist physicians and estheticians in adding esthetic skin-care services to the medical practice. The multifaceted issues that face the physician and the esthetician incorporating skin-care services can be somewhat overwhelming. Changes in the medical environment have prompted physicians to look for fee-for-service options in their practices. However, the busy physician may not have the time or perhaps the patience to explore all the business management, legal, and liability issues that would affect this type of relationship. Nor does the esthetician have the resources readily available to research this new growing area. Until now...

This book is a culmination of over eight years of experience and research in setting up over fifty practices across the United States and Canada. The laws vary widely, and I caution readers to check in their localities; however, the basic guidelines provided in this book should make the transition a little smoother!

Acknowledgments and Contributors

Catherine Atzen
Inga Ellzey
Linda Garofallou
Bea Franch-Hunter
Alison O'Neil
Paul Scott Premo
Susan Raef
Anna-Dee Rinehart
Ruth G. Sikes
Anne Willis
Sarah Wiskerchen

I also wish to acknowledge my research assistant, Richard A. Schlesinger, and my medical editor, Kathleen Kurtz.

❈ Contents ❈

CHAPTER ONE

Examining Your Career Options

Today's esthetician enjoys a broad range of career options. The esthetician can work in a traditional salon setting, either as an employee or as an independent contractor. He or she can choose a career in theatrical esthetics, working in makeup or hairstyling for the film industry, television, or the stage. And cosmetics companies offer numerous opportunities, from counter work in department stores to sales, management, and executive positions. All of these, however, lie outside the scope of this book, which is devoted to the role of the esthetician in medical settings.

In this chapter you will learn:

- the opportunities, advantages, and disadvantages of working as an esthetician in a medical practice

- what the work is like

- who is best suited for it

- the various kinds of practices that are most likely to use the services of an esthetician.

Is This the Kind of Work for Me?

Two questions should be considered when deciding whether to work in a medical setting: would I like it and would I be good at it? The answers may not be as obvious as you think.

1

Physicians and Estheticians
Share Many Characteristics

The reasons for choosing a career in medicine or in esthetics differ in many respects, but they also overlap in more ways than you might think, which makes combining the two a natural choice for some people.

People pursue careers in esthetics for various reasons. Obviously, one of the essentials is the enjoyment of working with people. There's really no room in the profession for people who don't genuinely enjoy dealing with others and helping them be their best. It takes real skill to put people at ease to the point where they trust us to keep their interests at heart. Often we have to learn to listen between the words to find out what clients really want, and estheticians frequently develop sophisticated psychological skills. Respecting our clients' privacy is important: remember the hair-coloring commercial that posed the question "Does she or doesn't she [today it could well be does he or doesn't he]? Only her hairdresser knows for sure!" The ad may sound old-fashioned, but the concept of respecting the trust people place in us is not.

We enjoy work that centers on our esthetic sensibility, and our training refines that sensibility and focuses it on helping people look their best. In a sense, ours is one of the so-called "helping professions," and as such, it has quite a bit in common with the other helping professions: part of the professional satisfaction comes from the knowledge that when a job is well done, we help someone.

Estheticians also like to work independently. That is, the esthetician is personally and directly responsible for the job he or she does. In a sense, that's true of just about any job, but some work, like ours, allows the person performing it to assume complete responsibility for the end results. If done well, the results are obvious, but their effects may be more subtle, revealing themselves in our clients' increased self-confidence. If done poorly, the results are equally obvious and the effects on our clients genuinely painful.

And let's not forget that we do it for the money.

In a lot of ways, what we've said about estheticians is equally true of physicians. The clinician, the physician actually engaged in patient care as opposed to research physicians, epidemiologists, and certain specialties such as pathology that often involve very little actual patient contact, must enjoy dealing with people. Physicians need to be able to put people at ease and win their trust. The Hippocratic oath that all physicians take when they get their medical degrees demands that the physician put the interests of the patient first and that the physician be governed by what is best for the patient, sometimes sacrificing self-interest. And the good physician respects his or her patients, always guarding their privacy and the confidential nature of the relationship.

Physicians to a large extent also enjoy working on their own. They value their independence, although that aspect of medicine is often threatened today by the movement toward cost-containment, health maintenance organizations (HMO), and various other forms of managed care. But it remains true that the physician is, to a degree often greater than others, personally responsible for the work he or she does. The consequences of doing the work well or poorly, especially in certain specialties, can be dramatic, literally life or death. But the day-to-day work is usually more mundane, although the impact on patients' lives is obviously enormous.

Physicians in certain specialties, particularly dermatology and plastic surgery, often have highly developed aesthetic sensibilities. In fact, quite a number of plastic surgeons are amateur artists, and sometimes more than amateur. After all, their work is to literally sculpt the human face and body.

And while the greatest reward is knowing that you've helped your patients, physicians, too, do it for the money.

A Matter of Ego

Now, let me state one thing. In comparing the esthetician with the physician, I don't mean to equate the two. In terms of education and training, there's no comparison. The physician generally spends a minimum of eight years beyond college, and frequently longer, in training. Physicians continue their formal education throughout their working lives and spend countless hours on their own reading journals, attending conferences, watching technical videos, and generally keeping abreast of developments in medicine and in their specialties. Estheticians also need to keep up with their field, but not to the same extent as physicians—either in importance or in the time spent.

In fact, this is a topic we'll be coming back to frequently in this book: what is the role of the esthetician in a medical setting in relation to the roles of the other people, professional and nonprofessional. From a legal standpoint, which we'll discuss at length in Chapter Six, "Insurance and Liability Issues," you should be absolutely clear about exactly what you can and can't do. But it's also important for estheticians considering working with physicians to understand that establishing professional limits and clearly defined roles is sometimes difficult but absolutely necessary if the personal and working relationship between physician and esthetician is to be a mutually satisfying one.

For now, it is enough to say that the esthetician brings to the medical practice expertise in skin care that the physician does not have and that can play a vital role in the physician's practice, especially in specialties such as dermatology and plastic and reconstructive surgery. At the same time, it's important to understand that egos—yours and the physician's—are involved in any working relationship, and the esthetician is almost always subordinate to the physician in a medical setting. That's as it should be from a medical standpoint. After all, the physician is first concerned with the patient's life and medical condition. How the patient looks comes second.

Why do I bring this up in the first chapter? Because, when examining your career options and deciding whether you really want to work in a medical context, you need to consider whether you're the kind of person who needs to be dominant in all situations. While the esthetician working in a medical setting *is* the expert in his or her sphere, that sphere is secondary to medical issues, and ultimately the physician is the boss. How much independence you achieve in a medical practice will depend on the relationship you work out with the physician(s) you work with, but in the final analysis you'll never have the kind of authority in a medical setting you would enjoy in a salon, especially if you own the salon. As usual, the first step in making a career decision is taking a good, honest look at yourself.

This Isn't "General Hospital"—It's the Real Thing

One of the most important factors in deciding whether to work in a medical setting is whether you like medicine. Specifically, are you comfortable dealing with illness and medical problems on a daily basis? The fields you're likely to choose shouldn't bring you into contact with many sick people, but your clients will all be patients, and all of them will have medical concerns. And while dermatology and plastic surgery, the areas you're most likely to work in, generally involve less serious medical problems, they're still not for the squeamish. Plastic surgery, after all, is still surgery. And some plastic surgeons perform reconstructive surgery to repair the trauma of accidents or the disfigurement of diseases such as cancer or genetic defects. Dermatologists treat skin cancer, burns, various rashes and infections, which can be disfiguring, as well as various diseases that affect the skin.

If you can't stand the sight of blood or if you find illness or disability overwhelming, then you probably shouldn't work in a medical setting. On the other hand, most of us can get used to the sights and the situations that are likely to come up in dermatology or plastic surgery, and if you are drawn to helping others and appreciate the privilege of working intimately with people who depend on you, the rewards of working in a medical setting can be tremendous.

What Do Estheticians Do in a Medical Practice?

What do estheticians working in a medical setting actually do? This book is not a text of "medical" esthetics, but I think it's appropriate to outline in broad terms what procedures an esthetician working in a medical practice is likely to do. The work can be divided into two broad categories: preparing the skin for medical procedures or surgery and teaching patients to take better care of their skin or effectively camouflage scars or other abnormalities.

Preparing the Skin for Medical Procedures

One of the most important roles you'll play in a medical setting is helping to prepare patients for surgery or other medical procedures. Estheticians are experts in cleansing and other techniques that create the best possible conditions for the skin; in fact, they frequently know more and have more experience in this area than physicians. Each physician will have his or her own protocol for preparing patients for surgery, but the general procedure tends to be the same. For facial cosmetic surgery, the regimen frequently begins three to six weeks prior to surgery with a thorough, deep cleansing of the face or neck, including exfoliation if the treatment is performed far enough in advance of the surgery. Treatments may be repeated at set intervals until about two weeks before surgery. The esthetician will also advise the patient about what makeup he or she can use during the weeks just before surgery. The object is to keep the skin as healthy as possible.

After surgery, the esthetician may perform various procedures designed to hasten healing, such as hydration and possibly lymphatic drainage, but actual manipulation of the skin is usually avoided until the skin and underlying tissue has had time to "set." When healing has progressed to the point where gentle manipulation can be performed, the esthetician will give the patient new makeup and instruction on how to apply it and how to keep the skin clean and healthy. Here's where your artistry will be important. Cosmetic techniques the patient relied on before surgery may no longer be appropriate, either because a problem the patient had tried to cover up no longer exists or because the lines and contours of the face have changed. Usually, the patient who's just had cosmetic surgery has a new interest in his or her new appearance and will turn to you for advice about products and techniques that make the most of it. You will, in essence, be responsible for putting the finishing touches on the whole experience.

For the reconstructive patient, the esthetician's expertise will again serve to make the most of the medical procedure. Special care may be needed to promote healing and minimize scarring, but the most important aspect of your work is often the skilled use of makeup to camouflage scarring or discoloration. Again, you will be called on to offer advice on which products and techniques are best. You will also be best qualified to design makeup that enhances new contours and draws attention to the patient's most attractive features. Remember, the deepest scars for the accident patient or the burn survivor may be the psychological ones that persist long after healing is complete. As the esthetician, you can play a very significant role in healing and even eliminating those scars.

Your role in a dermatologist's practice will be similar, although the focus may be more on helping patients develop good skin hygiene practices and avoiding makeup and cosmetic practices that compromise the skin. Under the physician's guidance, you will be responsible for extraction of comedomes, exfoliation, and ,when appropriate, light chemical peels. Chapter 2 goes into more detail on the types of services and procedures that you will be doing in a medical setting. You'll also advise the patient on avoiding comedogenic products and in recommending appropriate cosmetics. Patients may need help designing makeup to accommodate temporary discoloration of the skin due to illness or dermatologic procedures, or you may have to design camouflage to mask permanent conditions. You'll also advise patients, again under the physician's supervision, about how to avoid sun damage, which products are irritating or allergenic, and how to care for common acne and acne-related conditions. Reinforcing the patient's home-care routines, including proper usage of topical and oral medications, will also be an important role you will play in a dermatology practice.

Dermatology or Plastic Surgery

If you're serious about considering a career in "medical" esthetics, several paths are open to you. While a number of medical specialties can use the services of an esthetician, the most common are **dermatology** and **plastic surgery**. These are the two areas that deal most directly with skin appearance and aesthetics, and they offer the most opportunities for the esthetician. Let's spend a few minutes examining the scope of each specialty.

Dermatology

Dermatologists specialize in diseases of the skin, and in treating diseases, injuries, and genetic conditions that affect the skin, hair, and nails. Their training consists of a minimum of four years of college, four years of medical school, generally a year of internship in general medicine, and two to four years of specialty residency in dermatology. After completing their residency, dermatologists are eligible to take their board examinations in dermatology, administered by the American Academy of Dermatology. Once they pass this exam, which consists of written and practical or clinical portions, they can call themselves board-certified dermatologists.

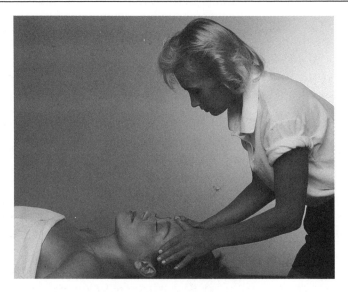

Estheticians often find opportunities in dermatology practices.

Some dermatologists train further to sub-specialize. They may specialize in general dermatologic surgery or in micrographic surgery (MOHS), which is used to treat certain skin cancers. Some dermatologists are now offering more cosmetic surgical procedures such as laser resurfacing and tumescent liposuction.

Other dermatologists specialize in cosmetic dermatology. These physicians often limit their practices to treating purely cosmetic disorders of the skin, hair, and nails or the cosmetic symptoms of other more generalized diseases, which are themselves treated by other physicians.

Plastic Surgery

The other medical specialty most likely to use the services of an esthetician is plastic surgery. The word *plastic* comes from the Greek word that means to mold, and plastic surgery literally molds, or remolds, the human body. There are two basic forms of plastic surgery: cosmetic surgery and reconstructive surgery.

Surgery is considered strictly cosmetic when it is performed solely for esthetic purposes, to make the patient look better. Among the more frequently performed cosmetic procedures are facelifts, nasal surgery, chin surgery, eyelid surgery, and breast augmentation or reduction. While this type of surgery is not medically necessary, it may be necessary for patients' psychological well being. In fact, the psychological dimensions of cosmetic surgery are sometimes almost as important as the physical ones; the payoff for this kind of surgery in enhanced self-confidence, socially and professionally, can be tremendous. Estheticians are particularly sensitive to the role that physical appearance can play in a person's life.

Reconstructive surgery, of course, is quite different, although often the object is similar. Burn patients, accident victims, people who have had major cancer surgery, and people born with deformities often need reconstructive surgery to restore functions that have been lost or to allow normal function that was absent at birth. Often the surgery also serves to restore a normal or near-normal appearance.

While many plastic surgeons perform both kinds of surgery, others specialize in one or the other. For the esthetician, the choice may come down to the kinds of patients you enjoy working with. Patients requiring reconstructive surgery have emotional needs that can be quite different from those of the patient who elects cosmetic surgery. For reconstructive surgery patients, esthetics may be secondary to the primary purpose for surgery, usually the restoration or preservation of function. The esthetician can play an important part in a reconstructive surgery practice. Preoperative skin care, helping the skin heal postoperatively, and using camouflage to minimize the cosmetic effects of the surgery play a vital role in restoring patients' confidence and well-being. But not everyone is comfortable dealing with people in pain on a daily basis.

On the other hand, reconstructive surgery can literally transform people's lives, and being a part of that kind of work can be extremely fulfilling. And for certain reconstructive procedures, the esthetic aspects can be absolutely central. Surgery for burn survivors and abused women, for instance, can go far toward restoring the elasticity of the damaged tissue and the contours that may have been lost, but it's rare that the appearance of the skin can be completely restored by surgery alone. The skilled use of makeup can frequently extend the effects of the surgical procedure, by restoring the appearance to what it was before the accident.

Independent Contractor or Employee; Full- or Part-Time; My Office or Yours?

Once you've decided on working in a medical setting, you still have to choose in what context you're going to do it. Right now, you have several options: you can work full- or part-time for a physician as part of a practice; or you can work in your own salon, seeing clients who are referred by the physician with whom you have an association. Each arrangement has its own advantages and drawbacks.

Many estheticians work full- or part-time in a physician's office as an employee. As such, the esthetician becomes part of the medical and professional team that follows patients from the first evaluative appointment through postoperative care in the case of plastic surgeons, or the resolution of a medical problem in the case of dermatologists. This arrangement provides the greatest immersion in the medical practice and generally offers the best opportunities for learning. It also often means taking on duties and responsibilities that may have little to do with your actual work as an esthetician. You might be responsible, for instance, for scheduling appointments for pre- and postoperative skin treatments and coordinating those appointments with the other visits the patient needs; you might be involved in billing for your services; you might be responsible for patient education; and you might have to share general administrative duties, such as manning a reception desk, with other people in the office.

The advantage of this situation is that you are treated as one of the team. As an employee, you can expect to receive the same fringe benefits that other employees get, including insurance coverage, paid vacation, reimbursement for continuing education, especially as it relates to your work, and, in some cases, participation in a retirement fund.

If you tend to be entrepreneurial, however, you may prefer to establish yourself as an **independent contractor**. This arrangement can offer many of the advantages we've just discussed, but without the fringe benefits. At the same time, it also means that you'll be responsible for running your own business. You'll have to pay your own taxes on a quarterly basis and pro-

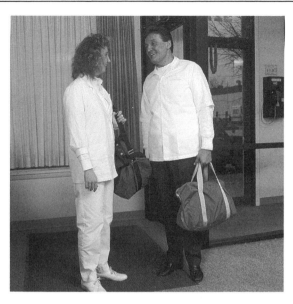

Working as an employee in a physician's office offers many advantages. It provides the greatest immersion in the medical practice and generally offers the best opportunities for learning.

vide for your own medical and disability insurance, and in some cases for malpractice insurance (more about that in Chapter Six). You may also need the services of an accountant and a lawyer to help set up your business. If you already have your own business, of course, you know what I'm talking about. But if you've never worked this way before, you should think carefully about whether you want to take on these business-related concerns.

The other option for estheticians who want to become more involved in a medical practice is to develop a referral business with a physician while continuing to work in a salon setting. Under this arrangement, a plastic surgeon, for instance, would refer patients to you for preoperative skin treatments and for postoperative follow-up care and instruction. This kind of arrangement is good for the esthetician who wants to explore working in a medical context but who is not yet committed to it full time. It allows you to try a new field without giving up your salon work. But don't make the mistake of thinking you'll just be adding a few more clients to your schedule; clients referred by the physician will take more of your time, especially in the

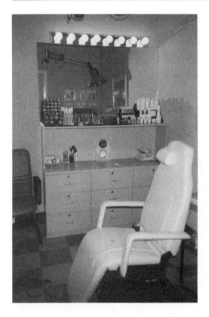

Another option for estheticians is to develop a referral business with a physician, for preoperative skin treatments and postoperative follow-up care and instruction.

beginning. You'll have to spend time with the physician learning what he or she expects for a given condition or procedure and learning the history and medical needs of each patient you'll be working with.

The next new area for estheticians will be to work directly in a hospital or rehabilitative center. At the moment, I'm not aware of any such positions, but I'm convinced it's only a matter of time before they open up. It makes sense for the same reasons that it makes sense for physicians to add our services to their practices: we provide additional value to patients and we open up additional sources of revenue that hospitals and other health facilities will find hard to ignore. In fact, if you have an entrepreneurial flair, you might approach your local hospital or rehabilitation center with a proposal to add esthetic services. Someone will do it. Why not you?

❦ Review and Summary ❦

For a growing number of estheticians, working with a physician is an attractive alternative or supplement to salon work. Working in a medical setting can be exciting and intellectually stimulating, and it can bring rewards that simply aren't available in any other context. But it isn't for everyone.

The options available to you as an esthetician and the reasons for choosing a career in a medical practice are the first considerations in deciding whether this career is for you. It is important to remember that the esthetician may bring to the medical practice a new area of expertise in skin care and cosmetics and play a vital role in the education of the patient, including pre- and postoperative care.

You can maintain independence in a medical practice while working with physicians. Always remember that the physician has the ultimate authority in patient care. The types of procedures performed in a medical practice by the esthetician vary widely. However, treatments performed in a medical practice differ from those in a salon or spa environment.

In a dermatology practice you deal with diseases of the skin such as acne, atopic dermatitis, and psoriasis. In a plastic surgery practice you deal with the pre- and postoperative care of the patient, perhaps performing lymphatic drainage, wound care, and advising the physician on the psychological status of the patient relating to the outcome of the surgery. The esthetician may also work with trauma patients or burn survivors, which can be very fulfilling. Esthetic treatments in a medical practice can go a long way in restoring the elasticity of damaged tissue and, through the skillful use of makeup, help to restore the self-image of the patient.

You have to decide on whether to work as an employee, full-time or part-time, in the physician's office or in your own private clinic. Several issues are related to this decision. Working as an employee can open up a variety of benefits that would not be available to you as an a sole proprietor. The benefits could be insurance coverage, vacation, continuing education, and participation in some type of retirement fund. However, if you work on a referral basis you would be responsible for the remainder of your taxes, planning for your retirement, and all the paperwork that goes with owning your own business.

Ask yourself the following questions:

- Am I comfortable dealing with people who may be ill, frightened, or in pain?

- Do I need always to be independent and in charge, or can I work comfortably in a team?

■ Am I willing to devote the time it takes to understand medical procedures and review patient cases?

■ Am I willing to take on tasks and responsibilities that go beyond the role of esthetician.

(If the answers to these questions is "yes", it may be time to think about what kind of medical practice you would like to be associated with and in what capacity.)

■ Do I prefer dermatology or plastic surgery, cosmetic or reconstructive surgery?

■ Do I want to do medical work full time or as a supplement to traditional esthetic work?

■ Should I be an employee or take referrals in my salon?

Becoming an esthetician in a physician's practice offers many rewards: the sheer excitement and intellectual stimulation that comes from stretching your skills and expanding the scope of your work; the knowledge that you've helped someone overcome a handicap or disability; being the one to put the finishing touches on a complex, highly skilled cosmetic surgical procedure.

Chapter Two

Esthetic Treatments in a Medical Setting

The addition of esthetic services to a medical practice requires planning, not only for marketing new services, but also for the additional training needed for the esthetician. **Esthetician training** varies from state to state, so the number of hours spent learning will depend on the location, ranging from 120 hours in some states to 600 hours in others. The separation of the esthetic license from the standard cosmetology or hairdressing license has allowed some schools to become licensed to teach only skin care, thereby raising their hours and standards.

Under the current regulations, I believe estheticians do not receive enough training, especially in the areas of anatomy, physiology, and chemistry, to fully understand the types of esthetic treatments that are beneficial in the medical practice. In this chapter we will explore services that have already proven to be successful in the medical setting and also new treatments that show great promise.

The most important point to remember before embarking on this new career path is that treatments that you are presently giving in the salon differ from those that you would provide in a medical office. You will have an opportunity to see more skin diseases, surgical procedures, and perhaps participate in trauma intervention and burn care.

Later chapters will discuss business issues, such as malpractice liability, insurance reimbursement, and marketing, but for

15

now just understand that working in a medical practice will require you to work harder, study longer, and continually read to educate yourself on the latest developments in the practice area.

In this chapter you will learn:

- the additional training you may need to work in a medical practice

- the stages of wound healing and how to monitor the postsurgical patient

- types of treatment masks that may be beneficial

- burn care and the complications that may face the burn survivor

- the causes and treatment of acne

- the benefits of lymphatic drainage in the pre- and postsurgical patient

- the role of the esthetician in the pre- and postoperative care of the patient

- helpful tips on cosmetic application for the surgical patient

Lymphatic Drainage Massage

Linda Garofallou

Lymph is a vital fluid that flows through the body in an intricate network of branching vessels and nodes. Essential for health and life, the lymphatic system plays a crucial role in the body's immune reactions and the processes of elimination. It participates in the process of nutrition and regeneration. In its nutritional role, the lymph conveys nutritive substances from the digestive tract into the bloodstream. Then, after these substances are metabolized, the lymph system helps to ferry the metabolic wastes from the cells, removing excess fluids, larger protein molecules, and pieces of damaged cells or extruded blood cells from the tissue spaces and returning them to the circulatory system.[1]

Manual **lymphatic drainage massage** is a hands-on technique that enhances the movement of lymph and connective tissue fluids in the body and promotes the normal, healthy functioning of the lymphatic system. A highly specialized set of massage techniques designed to promote the movement of lymphatic fluids was developed in the early 1930s by Emil and Estrid Vodder. This technique came to be known as Dr. Vodder's Manual Lymph Drainage (MLD). While there are several forms of lymphatic drainage massage in the world today, all owe their origins to the work of the Vodders. MLD has been widely employed in Europe, where the technique is practiced in hospitals and clinics. It is recognized by the Austrian and German government health insurance plans and is the third most prescribed physical therapy technique in Germany. Only recently has the technique become more widely known and practiced in the United States.

Manual Lymphatic Drainage Method

Dr. Vodder's MLD technique employs four basic hand movements: stationary circles, pumping, scooping, and rotary techniques.[2] Stationary circles use the palmar surface of the hands or the pads of the fingers to contact the skin and move it in continuous spiral movements. This technique is used primarily on the neck and face. Pumping and scooping techniques are used primarily on the arms and legs, while the more complex rotary movements are used on the large, flat surfaces of the body, such as the thorax, back, and abdomen.

Each of these four techniques specifically conform to the anatomy and physiology of the lymphatic system. The direction of the massage always follows the flow of the lymph in the body. Because forty percent of the body's lymph resides in the superficial layers of the skin,[3] the technique moves only the skin, not the underlying tissues. Since lymph naturally moves through a series of valved lymph vessels in a rhythmic, peristalic-like action, it is important to maintain this same rhythmic quality in the technique, using a stretch and release type of pumping movement. The degree of pressure must be very light and should be adjusted to suit the condition of the tissue. The more distended the tissue, the lighter the touch. Too much pressure can cause a dilated lymph vessel to collapse,[4] impeding the flow; however, too little pressure or the wrong type of movement will prove to be ineffective. A light, slow, intermittent, and rhythmic pumping action mirrors the body's own lymphatic movement and stimulates specific receptors in the skin that enhance lymph flow.

Treatments last fifteen to twenty minutes for the face and neck. The treatment for the body normally lasts sixty to ninety minutes, depending on the condition being treated.

Indications

Lymphatic drainage massage, when performed correctly by a trained and experienced person, is highly effective. Its effect on the sympathetic and parasympathetic nervous systems is both calming and soothing. By stimulating the stretch receptors surrounding the lymph vessels, lymph flow is increased, creating a decongestive effect on the loose connective tissue and increasing the resorptive capacity of the blood capillaries. This increases tissue drainage and helps eliminate edema and ecchymosis (bruising). Increasing lymph flow also has an immunological effect. It increases the activity of the lymphocytes, allowing them to more readily come into contact with antigens. Pathogenic substances are then rapidly transported to the lymph nodes, where they can be rendered harmless. Finally, MLD has an analgesic effect, stimulating inhibitory receptors, which can decrease or eliminate pain sensations.

There are numerous indications for lymphatic drainage massage. It is very effective when used in conjunction with esthetic facial treatments in helping to maintain clean, toned, and healthy skin. The indications for dermatologic conditions include acne, telangiacstasis, rosacea, and noninflammatory atopic dermatitis. MLD is very beneficial for traumatic injuries that result in swelling and bruising, making it particularly effective for postsurgical edema and hematoma. In addition to these indications, considerable scientific and clinical data point to its effectiveness in the treatment of postmastectomy lymph edema, scar tissue,[5] and chronic inflammatory disorders such as arthritic swelling, bursitis, and tendinitis.

As with any therapeutic modality it is most important to obtain proper training and experience before attempting to use the method in a treatment setting. Lymphatic drainage massage cannot be learned by reading a book or article in a magazine. Training should include education in the scientific basis of the method, in anatomy and physiology, as well as in practical instruction of the method.

Contraindications

Manual lymph drainage is contraindicated in the following conditions:

1. All malignant diseases

2. Any acute inflammatory condition with infection

3. Thrombosis

4. Cardiac edema

5. Hypotension

6. Certain metabolic disorders, such as thyroid disease

Conclusion

Due to the subtleties in its functioning and in its anatomy, the lymphatic system has, throughout history, been the subject of much neglect, misunderstanding, and controversy. Recent technological advances and specialized techniques have finally made this elusive network accessible to study, resulting in great advances in our understanding of this incredibly complex system. Scientific research has demonstrated[6] the effectiveness of the movements of the lymphatic drainage technique.[7] At the same time, clinical observations have shown its beneficial effects. The intimate relationship between the lymph system and the health of the skin, through the lymph's renewal of connective tissue fluid, activation of circulation, stimulation of cell activity, and the regeneration of facial tissue, make lymphatic drainage massage of the face and neck an essential tool in every medical esthetic practice.

Lymphobiology® Treatments

Catherine Atzen

A lymphatic drainage treatment was developed that uses a machine providing pulsed suction to expedite the lymph; the method is called **Lymphobiology®**. Lymphobiology® treatments are used for improvement in the skin's condition, wrinkles, elasticity of the skin, and reduction in sensitivity. Lymphobiology® is a registered trademark of Catherine Atzen Laboratories in Campbell, California.

Lymphobiology® Benefits

Preoperative: three sessions of Lymphobiology® will improve the texture and elasticity of the skin and eliminate lymph stasis (which causes swelling).

Postoperative: five sessions will be performed starting the day after surgery, resulting in:

- a reduction in edema and ecchymosis,
- an acceleration of cyclid healing,
- reduction of rhytids,
- reduction of the patient's discomfort related to postoperative edema,
- a lowering of the sympathetic nervous system, which is relaxing to the patient.

Safety and Efficiency

Lymphobiology® has an outstanding track record for safety and efficiency.

An estimated 15,000 persons have benefited from this treatment.

Results and feedback from patients and physicians are extremely positive.

Medical Studies

Lymphobiology® is a therapeutic procedure for the pre- and postoperative periods, substantiated by a double blind study on patients undergoing blepharoplasty.

During the double blind study, only one side of the face was treated.

Ninety percent of the patients showed a major improvement in the healing process: diminishing of rhytids (wrinkles), edema (swelling), and ecchymosis (bruising on the treated side).

Patients also feel less discomfort.

Procedure

1. Cleanse and use toner.

2. Massage 1/4 flask Integral DNA b.e.® until complete penetration.

3. Apply cream generously.

4. Attach the glass tubes, and turn on the equipment.

5. The procedure is done following this pattern: start sliding tubes along the sternocleidomastoid area and cover the entire neck, finishing each movement at the subclavian vein.

6. Follow with chin and jawline area.

7. Then do the face area (medial area first).

8. Next is the eye area and forehead.

9. Rinse off any excess cream.

10. Reapply toner.

11. Massage 1/4 flask Integral DNA b.e.® until complete penetration.

12. Moisturize and use sunblock as recommended.

Important for Postoperative Patients

The tubes need to remain 1 inch away from any incision, and the esthetician should not touch an incision or apply products on it until the skin has healed.

Turn the equipment to its lowest power for postoperative clients.

Communicate with the physician.

Follow the exact procedure as directed by the developer of the treatment. Training for this treatment is available and takes about one day.

Only use products recommended in the manufacturer's procedure.

Using Masks in the Medical Setting

Alison O'Neil

Throughout the development of the field of esthetics in the medical practice, the use of treatment masks as an integral part of skin treatments has been questioned. Results from masks are recognized as short term and therefore less important than other topical medications, which are left on the skin and repeatedly applied for long-term results. **Masks** are cosmetic products designed with concentrated oil-drying or hydrating product bases, such as clays, gels, or lotions, which are frequently blended with active medicated ingredients designed for temporary treatment.

The Purpose of Masks

Masks are designed to temporarily treat a variety of skin conditions. Products differ in their active ingredients, concentration, and composition. Estheticians are guided in the use of masks by the condition(s) to be treated. Some facial masks are helpful in sebum absorption, comedolytic action, or healing. Masks are also noted for their ability to help hydrate the skin when used postoperatively for wound healing. Masks may act as a brief intervention to correct the inability of the skin to hold water, known as transepidermal water loss (TEWL). Masks complement the patient's daily home-care program, and their use promotes healthier skin.

Masks for Acneic Skin

The use of a treatment mask may precede the invasive procedure of acne surgery and be used postsurgically, for anti-inflammatory purposes, depending on the clinical observations of the esthetician. The purpose of a mask used prior to acne surgery is to soften and remove the stratum corneum, which blocks the opening of the follicle, in order to ensure less trauma during the procedure or to further promote a bacteria-free environment. The most common "active" ingredients found in masks for acneic skin include sulfur, **resorcinol, benzoyl peroxide**, and salicylic acid. When designed for acneic or oily skin, these ingredients are generally combined with vehicles known for their drying and oil-absorbing qualities, such as the clay substances **bentonite** and **kaolin**.

Sulfur alone or combined with resorcin has some anti-bacterial effect and is therefore helpful in healing acne lesions. These ingredients may also have some effects on normalizing follicular keratinization. Although benzoyl peroxide and sulfur are considered safe when used independently of one another, when combined, the sulfur is said to increase the possibility of sensitization to the benzoyl peroxide.

Salicylic acid, although not as effective as tretinoin, acts directly on the follicle, thereby helping to unblock plugged hair follicles. Most importantly, it can help prevent new comedo development because of its effect on the abnormal desquamation process (skin cell

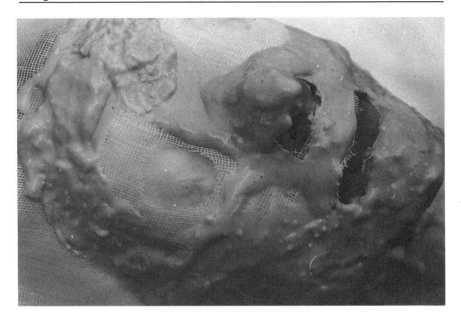

Patient in a clay mask

shedding rate). Salicylic acid is most beneficial for mild cases of acne identified by the presence of multiple small comedos or blackheads.

To avoid unnecessary skin irritation, the length of exposure to products containing active ingredients should be closely monitored. Furthermore, the esthetician should remain with the patient throughout this intervention, since the patient may not recognize signs of sensitivities. Signs of irritation include redness, burning, itching, or stinging. If any of these signs exist it should be treated, noted in the patient's chart, and the patient should be made aware of the sensitivity to avoid any future problems.

Hydrating Masks

Hydrating masks may have effects lasting for up to a few days. Masks designed to hydrate skin are generally thicker in texture. **Hydrating masks** contain thickening agents such as titanium dioxide, gelling agents, or ingredients that chemists call "thickeners." Additionally, the most common "active" ingredients used in masks for rehydration include:

1. **humectants** which attract water,

2. **emollients** which help to temporarily plump up small lines and wrinkles,

3. extracts from plants, which can act as humectants or as irritants, creating the temporary effect again of plumping fine lines and wrinkles,

4. other "specialized conditioning" agents, which are available to chemists.

Although there is less likelihood of sensitization to ingredients contained in moisturizing masks, the esthetician should always note any known skin sensitivities, inhalant allergies, family history of eczema, and any previous contact or atopic dermatitis. Some patients may be allergic to preservatives, fragrances, and color used in many cosmetic products. To avoid potential reactions, choose simple products containing little to no color or fragrance, therefore limiting exposure to the most likely irritant preservatives. Note: Products labeled as "natural" are not necessarily preservative free.

Most masks designed for hydration of the epidermis feel soothing. Clay and gel masks are presumed to stimulate the underlying blood flow and aid in superficial cleansing of tissue. This is indeed what they do, but it is of little or no benefit to aging skin. These masks cannot enliven aging skin or cause degenerating fibrous tissue to rejuvenate into youthful elasticity. Pores cannot permanently "shrink or close", and the feeling of tightness that occurs is transient. However, hydrating masks may have some uncalculated yet beneficial effect on wound healing when used pre- and postoperatively on facial surgery patients.

Although there is much data available regarding both the potential effectiveness and side effects of the active ingredients mentioned above, the introduction of esthetic treatments in a medical setting is still new, and formal clinical studies have not been completed that would quantitatively prove the overall benefits of masks. The use of masks has been perpetuated in large part by the sharing of "success" stories among estheticians. There is also the very real psychological benefit of relaxation, which has resulted in the continued use of masks as an integral part of at-home facial care.

It is important to note that some of the mask products available require close monitoring. Within the clinical setting,

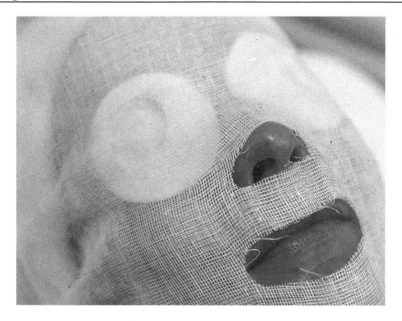

Client with gauze and eye pads covering the face

knowledge of the patient's history and current medical treatments plays a key role in the overall success or failure of the selected treatment program. The physician's orders must always be taken into account. Patients may be taking a medication such as **Accutane®** (an oral medication used for cystic acne), where, for instance, skin that was once oily and resilient is now dehydrated and fragile. Choosing the mask should therefore complement and be coordinated with the physician's prescribed treatment.

Wound Care

Anne Willis

The responsibility of an esthetician who treats surgical, trauma, and burn patients may include the need to monitor wounds and their care. An esthetician does not directly treat wounds; this falls in the medical domain. However, knowledge of the stages of wound healing is essential. It is important to realize that even though an external wound is closed and healing well, the underlying wounds need to be approached with caution.

It is important that the esthetician is capable of identifying the etiology, depth, color, and size of a wound and the mechanism behind the actual capability the skin has to heal itself. The esthetician can act as a monitor between surgeon and patient by detecting or recognizing possible complications, and referring the patient back to the physician for prompt treatment.

Understanding the different stages of wound healing allows the esthetician to develop a time frame for administering the treatment and determining the specific treatment to be done.

Avoiding wounded skin because it looks and feels sore is incorrect. Injury to the skin is part of the surgical process. How the skin is treated before and after the procedure affects the overall outcome.

Identifying a Wound

A **wound** is a break in the continuity of soft parts of body structures caused by violence or trauma to tissues.

The color of a wound will either be red, yellow, or black. Hematomas or ecchymosis (bruising) can be many colors. Dermis normally will take one week to **epithelize**, healing with skin regrowth, if cared for properly. All wounds will initially appear red and may stay this color for several months, lightening to a soft pink. Red is an indication that the wound is healthy. Yellow indicates infection, and in some, but not all, cases, black can mean dead tissue or necrosis.

Wounded skin may also take on a blanched appearance, which could be the beginning stage of ischemia or delayed healing. This may occur due to the lack of blood supply. Blood supply may be compromised due to excess swelling, lack of good nutrition, or too much tension applied to the skin.

Wound Sizes

The size of a wound can determine whether or not the wound is healing properly. The smaller the wound remains during the healing process, the healthier the result. When a wound extends or expands beyond the initial break to the surface, it becomes vulnerable to infection.

Wounds After Surgery

When there is a tear or break to the surface of the skin, a wound is made. The repair and restoration process begins immediately.

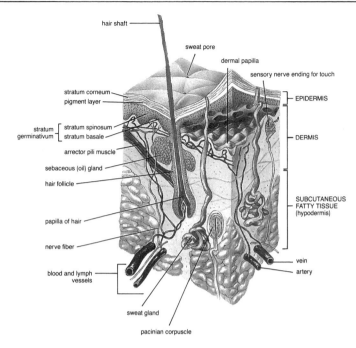

hair shaft

sweat pore

dermal papilla

sensory nerve ending for touch

stratum corneum
pigment layer

EPIDERMIS

stratum germinativum
stratum spinosum
stratum basale

DERMIS

arrector pili muscle

sebaceous (oil) gland

hair follicle

SUBCUTANEOUS FATTY TISSUE (hypodermis)

papilla of hair

nerve fiber

vein
artery

blood and lymph vessels

sweat gland

pacinian corpuscle

Cross section of the skin

Wounds occur after surgery, both externally and internally. External wounds are caused during the initial invasion of the skin, which is necessary to gain access to underlying muscle and fat. Internal wounds are made during the dissection of the dermis and the subcutaneous layer.

Stage One

The first stage is the intimation of the cellular process. **Polymorphs** (a type of white blood cell) and **macrophages** (phagocytic cells) play a key role in the protection and defense of the cut surface. **Platelets** clot to stop bleeding. It is vital to support these cells with proper nutrition both internally and externally.

Many estheticians specializing in wound recovery feel that lymphatic drainage treatment helps the patient heal more rapidly.

Stage Two

The second stage involves the introduction of fibroblasts. **Fibroblasts** are cells that crawl like spiders, leaving a web of collagen behind, allowing rearrangement of the connective tissue. If a wound is kept moist during this stage, a slippery foundation allows these spiderlike cells to work more efficiently. During this stage, the epidermis begins its initial migration over the wound edge.

Stage Three

A scab is formed, and the **myofibroblast** appears. A myofibroblast is a multiunit of cells that provide cell contraction. This contraction causes a force that draws the edge of the wound toward the center of the wound, thus closing it. During this process, the basal layer actively proliferates, forming a covering over the wound.

Stage Four

During stage four, completion of the epitheliazation of the exposed wound is accomplished. Contracting continues, strengthening the deeper layers of the wound. The scab is forced off by contraction, promoted by the myofibroblast. A scab should never be pulled off. It acts as a natural bandage, protecting the underlying wound. Removing a scab too soon may carry healthy tissue with it, which may lead to scarring. Generally, during stage four the esthetician may begin skin treatments.

Stage Five

The exterior wound is healed, the cut blood vessels are reunited, and new collagen reorganizes the underlying wound. This process may take up to one year to complete.

Wound Depths

The depth of the wound is commonly classified in three degrees, but it is measured more precisely in terms of the thickness of the injury.

A **first-degree**, or superficial, **wound** involves only the epidermis (top layer of the skin).

A **second-degree**, or partial thickness, **wound** involves the dermis as well as the epidermis.

A **third-degree**, or full-thickness, **wound** involves both layers of skin and the skin appendages—the hair follicles, sweat glands, sebaceous glands, and muscle is exposed.

Burn Care

Treatment for burns is based on location and depth, and therefore the topical medication utilized is burn specific. Regardless of the topical medication applied, the treatment goal is to prevent infection to the necrotic tissue. Some of the most common topical treatments for the burn patient include **Bacitracin®**, **Silver Sulfadiazine®**, **Sulfamylon®**, and **Silver Nitrate®**.[8]

Bacitracin® is a topical antibiotic used on superficial burns with a break in the epidermal layer. It is commonly used on all facial burns as it is less irritating to the eyes and therefore less painful. A thin layer should be applied utilizing sterile technique and reapplied as necessary to maintain a thin layer.

Silver Sulfadiazine® is a bactericidal for gram positive and negative organisms and yeast. This antimicrobial is used for second- and third-degree burns. Utilizing sterile technique, it is applied in a layer approximately a half to one inch thick. Recommended application is BID (twice daily) or as needed. This schedule maintains moisture in the wound and promotes natural debridement (sloughing of eschar). It cannot be used on a patient with silver and or sulfa allergies, and it has been noted to cause **leukopenia**, or a reduction in the number of leukocytes in the blood.

Sulfamylon® is also bacteriostatic for gram positive and negative organisms, especially pseudomonas. It will diffuse through devascularized tissue and is absorbed systematically. This systemic distribution may result in metabolic alkalosis (opposite of acidosis, which is extreme acidity of internal fluids in your vascular system). It is commonly used for areas of dense cartilage (ears) or severely infected wounds. However, it is not recommended for cartilage on the facial area (nose) because of increased irritation. Sulfamylon is also contraindicated in patients with a sulfa allergy.

Silver Nitrate® is an antibacterial agent used when a patient has a sulfa allergy or has had a leukopenic reaction to silver sulfadiazine. It is a sterile, wet dressing applied daily and should remain moist throughout the day. Silver nitrate has a tendency to stain the skin brown. To protect from staining, petroleum jelly should be applied to the healthy tissue of the burn periphery with each dressing change. Silver nitrate is not used as a first choice therapy.

If a third-degree burn is greater than twenty-five percent of the total body surface, auto-grafting and hospitalization is required. Postoperatively, these wounds are dressed with

Garamycin® gauze (anti-microbial dressing) to prevent infection. The donor site is a superficial, clean wound, which tends to heal within ten days. A hydrocolloid dressing remains in place until healing is complete.

Other Complications That May Occur in the Burn Survivor

- **Contractures.** Contractures result when scar tissue forms over or adjacent to a joint or skin fold. The shortened skin causes a loss of range of motion. These may be corrected through continued physical therapy, but may often require surgery.

- **Hypertrophic scars.** This ropey, thick formation of skin is an abnormal configuration of collagen fibers. The scars may be corrected with elastic pressure garments, steroid injection, or partial removal of the scar and regrafting. (Keloid formation is a special kind of scarring and is common to dark-pigmented skin).

- **Eye injuries.** Inability to close the eyes due to badly burned eyelids can be corrected with grafting. Scarring of the cornea often responds to medication, but a corneal transplant may be helpful.

- **Body part loss.** Amputations may be required if burns involve muscle and bone. The loss of the nose and ears is a fairly frequent complication and requires plastic surgery.

- **Neuromuscular problems.** Peripheral neuromuscular problems are evidenced by numbness, tingling, peripheral weakness, impaired hearing, or other nerve deficit signs. Hemiplegia, seizure disorders, aphasia, encephalitis, and meningitis have been found.

- **Loss of sweat glands.** The person must avoid overheating.

- **Hair loss.** A full-thickness burn involves the hair follicles, and thus the grafted areas will not grow hair. If the scalp is involved, hair transplants may be desired.

- **Loss of sebaceous glands.** Daily lubrication is needed to maintain pliable skin.

- **Delicate skin.** During the first year after grafting, even scratching can break the skin, and the skin will sunburn easily.

- **Itching.** Itching is a common complaint.

- **Lack of sensation.** Grafted areas lack the sensation of normal skin.

- **Drug dependency.** Whether this is a problem before or after injury, drug dependency complicates vocational planning.

Other serious complications are total loss of hearing and brain damage. Electrical burns merit special consideration. All electrical burns are full-thickness burns and usually occur at work. They often appear to involve only small areas where the current entered and exited, but the tissue beneath the skin may be severely damaged. This can lead to amputation and/or serious neuromuscular problems.[9]

Alpha-Hydroxy Acid (AHA) Cosmetic Exfoliation

Paul Scott Premo

The Esthetic Manufacturers/Distributors Alliance (EMDA) has developed professional guidelines for **alpha-hydroxy acid (AHA)** cosmetic chemical exfoliation procedures for cosmetologists and/or estheticians. The guidelines are intended to ensure procedural consistency in the use of professional rinse-off, pulse applications of alpha-hydroxy acids (glycolic and lactic) for which product safety has been substantiated. These guidelines exclude all other chemical exfoliation/peeling procedures and substances including, but not limited to, Jessner Peels, trichloracetic acid (TCA), carbolic acid (phenol), resorcinol, or combinations thereof.

Cosmetic chemical exfoliation procedures utilizing alpha-hydroxy acids facilitate stratum corneum desquamation, improving the esthetic appearance and quality of the skin. Cosmetic chemical exfoliation procedures are not intended to elicit viable epidermal and/or dermal wounding, injury, or destruction, and therefore differ from chemical peeling procedures administered by physicians. These guidelines cover "professional use only" AHA products (glycolic and lactic acids) with a concentration not exceeding thirty percent, pH 3.0, their application, precautions, and post-procedural care.

The following training program guidelines are recommended by the Esthetic Manufacturers/Distributors Alliance:

1. Scientific overview of alpha-hydroxy acids

2. Clinical indications vs. cosmetic applications

3. Client general history, skin evaluation, realistic expectations

4. Contraindications/precautions

5. Predisposition patch testing

6. Client preapplication care

7. Application procedure

8. Postapplication care

9. Client follow-up

Recommended Alpha-Hydroxy Acid (AHA) Cosmetic Chemical Exfoliation Procedure

1. Appropriate disinfection and sanitation, as established by respective state board of cosmetology.

2. Client preparation and protection, as established by respective state board of cosmetology.

3. Predisposition patch testing

   Sensitivity to chemical exfoliation products can only be determined by administering a predisposition patch test. This is recommended to be done twenty-four hours prior to the application of AHA cosmetic chemical exfoliating procedures.

4. Client consultation

   A thorough skin evaluation and consultation should be conducted on each client to determine if the procedure is appropriate.

   Suggested questions during the client consultation:

History of sun exposure and/or tanning bed use

History of cosmetic-related irritant/allergic contact dermatitis

Currently under physician's care

History of medication; i.e., tretinoin (Retin-A®, Renova®), isotretinoin (Accutane®, etc.)

HSV (herpes simplex virus) predisposition

Previous facial plastic/reconstructive surgery

Previous chemical exfoliation procedure—type and results

Current skin-care regimen including alpha-hydroxy acids

Precaution

A client history of cosmetic-related irritant/allergic reactions, HSV (cold sore) predisposition, current sun exposure or tanning bed use, and use of topical and/or oral medications may increase an individual's susceptibility to adverse reactions. Under these circumstances a predisposition patch test is recommended twenty-four hours before the procedure and/or physician advice. Cosmetic chemical exfoliation procedures are not recommended when a client is under the supervision of a physician for skin-related disorders, post chemical peel, laser treatment, or plastic/reconstructive surgery without the approval of the physician.

5. Client skin evaluation and inspection:

   A. Outline realistic expectations with client.

   It is not recommended to administer cosmetic chemical exfoliation procedures to skin exhibiting open cuts, sores, sunburn, chemical or thermal burns, or apparent skin irritation or sensitivity. Twenty-four hours prior to the procedure, a predisposition patch test is also recommended. Client photo documentation is also recommended at baseline and upon conclusion of each procedure.

   B. Thoroughly evaluate facial skin.

   C. Check for degree of sebaceous activity (skin oiliness), acne, telangiectasias (broken capillaries), photodamage, etc.

D. Check for open cuts, sores, lesions or apparent skin irritation or sensitivity.

6. Administering the cosmetic chemical exfoliation procedure:

The use of latex or vinyl gloves are recommended during the procedure.

Drape and protect client appropriately according to the established state board of cosmetology rules and regulations

Conduct client skin evaluation and inspection

Cleanse client's skin according to manufacturer's directions

Apply protective eye pads to eye area

Apply cosmetic chemical exfoliation preparation according to the recommended procedure of the manufacturer. The use of disposable implements is recommended.

Please note that manufacturer's directions can vary—always read carefully and follow complete directions.

■ Always follow manufacturer's directions regarding exposure time.

■ Remove preparation after the appropriate exposure time with cool, damp gauze or cotton pads.

■ Conclude procedure with manufacturer's skin-care procedure including the use of a UVA/UVB sunscreen or sunblock of SPF15.

■ Instruct client on any appropriate after-care.

■ Have client report to you any adverse reaction. Seek medical assistance if necessary.

■ Depending on the skin type and condition, it is recommended not to exceed two cosmetic chemical exfoliation procedures within one week, to a maximum of six.

The Esthetics Manufacturers/Distributors Alliance (EMDA) proposes this document as "recommended guidelines" for licensed cosmetologists/estheticians and professional beauty

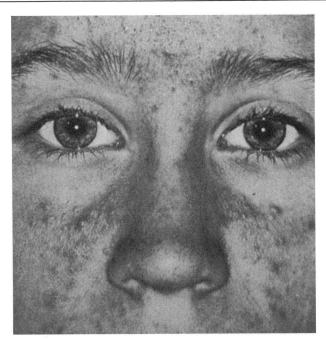

A patient with acne

manufacturers/distributors of alpha-hydroxy acid skin-care products and procedures and as such does not intend this document to supersede existing rules or regulations established by individual state boards of cosmetology or other local and state governing agencies.[10]

Acne Treatment

Acne vulgaris is the most common skin condition found in the second to third decades of life. More than eighty percent of adolescents develop some degree of acne.[11] This inflammatory disorder may leave scars, which are both physically and psychologically disabling. A new subset of patients with adult acne is emerging, where cosmetics and the role of androgens and stress may play a more significant role.

Four major factors that cause acne are

1. excess oil or sebum production;

2. abnormal follicular keratinization;

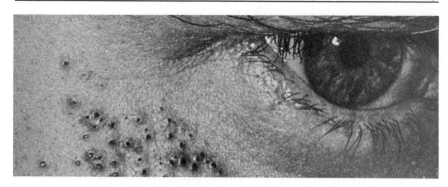

Comedones in the eye area

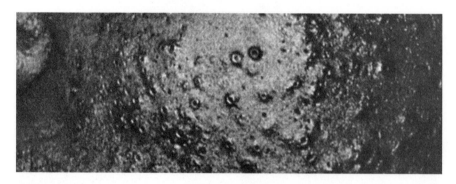

An ingrown hair

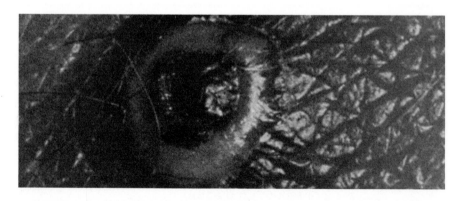

A pustule

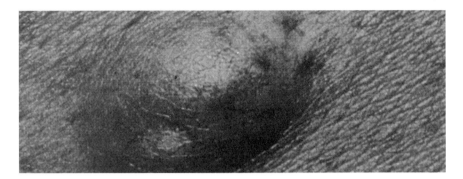

A cyst

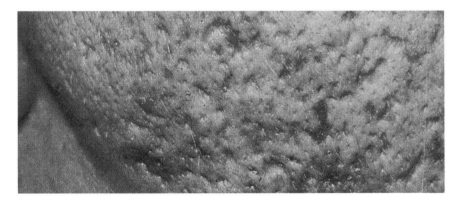

Acne scars

3. excessive proliferation of Propionibacterium acnes (*p. acnes*) in the hair follicle; and,

4. host factors, which include hormonal and immunologic considerations.

All treatment modalities are geared toward reducing sebum production, normalizing exfoliation, reducing *p. acnes*, and other factors mentioned previously. Topical agents are antibiotics, which suppress p. acnes and the resultant inflammation; tretinoin, which alters abnormal keratinization and is subsequently comedolytic; benzoyl peroxide, which acts as a peeling and antibacterial agent; and topical anti-inflammatory agents, such as sulfur and salicylic acid preparations, which have drying and anti-inflammatory properties. Systemic approaches include systemic antibiotics, oral isotretinoin, and hormonal therapy. Isotretinoin affects all four areas of pathophysiology, while estrogen and antiandrogens suppress sebum production.[12]

The **microcomedo** is the earliest precursor lesion of acne that may lead to inflammatory nodulocystic lesions. Extraction of comedones and incision and drainage of cysts has been shown to be helpful in preventing progression of inflammatory lesions and subsequent scarring.

The following treatment was utilized in a study involving 400 patients (200 in the study group and 200 in the control group) with a mean twelve-month follow-up. The study group consisted of 200 female patients with nodulocystic acne vulgaris. The patients underwent a regimen of monthly skin treatments (as outlined below); oral minocyline, 100 mg. twice a day; a topical regimen of 1 percent clindamycin lotion; a 4 percent benzoyl peroxide gel; a colloidal oatmeal soap; and a daily astringent. The results of the study suggested that a skin-care program utilizing skin treatments is helpful in treating patients with cystic acne. The study also concluded that the treatments, as outlined below, may actually decrease the patient's need for long-term systemic and topical agents.

Steps in the skin treatment program included

1. superficial cleansing;

2. exfoliation;

3. steaming;

4. acne surgery;

5. application of topical antibiotic (clindamycin);

6. an adjuvant anti-inflammatory agent, azelaic acid, applied to inflammatory lesions;

7. cool compressing;

8. application of SPF-8 nonacnegenic cream; and

9. intralesional triamcinolone injections (3 mg/cc) to inflammatory and cystic lesions in both the study and control groups, when indicated.

Conclusion

The treatment procedures that may be utilized in the medical setting to treat acne may vary from the treatment above and may include chemical agents to exfoliate the skin, liquid nitrogen "ice balls" to calm the skin after acne surgery, or the application of a sulphur-based mask. The practices of the physician and the esthetician may require a little rethinking in order to come up with acne treatment protocols that will satisfy them both.

Cryogenic Therapy

Bea Franch-Hunter

Cryogenic therapy, the therapeutic use of cold, has been used for over fifty years in dermatology to treat a variety of benign and neoplastic conditions.

Graded degrees of cold and various agents used are easily applied and usually require no anesthesia. Because the epidermal-dermal separation is above the basement membrane, there is no collagen destruction; therefore no scarring occurs after reepitheliazation.

Due to its rich vascular supply, skin is relatively resistant to freezing and acts as a good insulator. Injuries that do occur are directly proportional to the depth and intensity of freezing. A single freeze is less damaging than a repeated freeze-thaw application. The most intense injury is caused by a rapid cool-slow thaw application.

It is unclear exactly how the mechanism of injury works. Changes occur due to mechanical damage to the cells. As the nucleus is ruptured, the cell walls break down from ice formation and osmotic changes due to cellular dehydration, resulting in an increased number of electrolytes. Also, the lipid-protein complex in the cell membrane becomes denatured and tissue necrosis occurs due to vascular stasis.

The most popular agents used in dermatology are solid carbon dioxide (CO_2) at a boiling point of -78.5° C, and liquid nitrogen, at -195.6° C. Liquid nitrogen has become the standard therapeutic agent in cryosurgery because it is inexpensive, noncombustible, and is readily available. However, being the coldest agent available, liquid nitrogen can produce permanent skin damage by blistering.

In the field of medical skin care, CO_2 is gaining much popularity among estheticians. Less destructive than liquid nitrogen, CO_2 applications have many positive benefits for medical skin care correction and maintenance.

Benefits and Indications

Cryogenic therapy has many benefits. Dry ice therapy for the treatment of acne vulgaris has been utilized for many years. The procedure causes desquamation and involution of lesions. It is antibacterial and anti-inflammatory to the tissues and promotes healing. The use of cryogenic therapy does not prevent the formation of new acne lesions, but the vasoconstrictor effect reduces erythema, and the cooling action appears to tighten the pores, although this is transitory.

Other dermatologic indications and treatments include removal of warts, pigmented nevi, small keloid scars, seborrheic keratoses, and lentigines. Melanocytes are more sensitive to cold injury than keratinocytes and are selectively damaged by CO_2.

More recently, CO_2 has been utilized in the treatment of large areas of solar elastoses, lentigines, and actinic keratosis. The procedure eliminates damaged tissue and significantly reduces the potential for skin cancer. The stimulation of new cell growth increases cell turnover and plays a major role in the skin's rejuvenation process.

The best candidates for full face cryogenic therapy are patients with diffusely leathered skin, multiple actinic keratoses (pre-skin cancers), and solar elastoses. The treatment does not induce scarring and is safe for all skin types. Special caution must be used on sensitive skins, especially those who burn easily or have vascular conditions.

CO_2 should be used with caution on dark olive or ethnic skin types. The treatment can induce pigmentation abnormalities, especially if hard pressure is applied. Although permanent hypopigmentation and post-inflammatory hyperpigmentation are rare.

Preparation and Application

Dry ice may be purchased in several forms. Solid blocks of ice at a temperature of -78.5° C may be obtained from ice plants, food-packing plants, dairies, fishing bait supply stores, or pharmaceutical supply companies. It must be stored in a freezer or ice chest.

Protective gloves and eyewear should always be used. The blocks should be broken to hand-size pieces, wrapped in a small towel, and dipped in a 3:1 solution of acetone and alcohol to activate.

Carbon dioxide (CO_2) comes in a gas tank purchased through a welding supply company. The following of the Hazards Communication Standards and Occupational Safety and Health Act (OSHA) protocols are a must. Protective eyewear and gloves must be used while collecting and working with the gas. A leather chamois bag is wrapped around the nozzle of the tank. When the gas is released, it is captured in the bag, forming ice. The ice is then transferred to a stainless steel bowl, chopped fine with a pie blender, and prepared into balls. Hand packing the ice is very effective when used for superficial peeling.

Using a double layer of 4 x 4 and 2 x 2 opened gauze pads, the ice is placed in the center of the gauze, the corners are gathered together, and packed into balls. Ice balls may be stored in a thermal container for several hours at a time.

To activate the CO_2, dip the ice ball into acetone or acetone/alcohol mixture (3:1). Acetone dissolves sebum, converts the temperature of the CO_2 by accelerating the change from a solid to a gas form, and allows for easy slippage over the skin. Remove all slush that forms around the ice ball and bleeds through the gauze with a towel. Wipe clean until the ice is almost dry.

Keep the patient's eyes closed and well protected with goggles or pads at all times. Any flake of ice that gets into the eyes could result in corneal injury. Using even strokes, keep the CO_2 moving quickly over the entire surface of the skin with light pressure, especially over bony structures. The depth of penetration is determined by two factors:

1. the amount of saturation in acetone and dryness of the ball;

2. the amount of pressure applied during the application process.

CO_2 should never be allowed to sit on the skin for more than a split second. Skin reaction ranges from mild erythema to vesiculobullae formation. Solid CO_2 can produce complete epidermal necrosis in the stratum corneum when applied to the skin for fifteen seconds with hard pressure. This superficially aggressive modality should only be performed by a physician to treat specific skin disorders.

For acne patients following acne surgery, tap each lesion lightly several times, for a split second only. This will kill the remaining bacteria on the lesion and accelerate the healing process. Finish the treatment with an application of a topical antibiotic, such as erythromycin or clindamycin.

Cryogenic therapy is a stimulating, healing, regenerating treatment modality that can be a beneficial alternative for patients who are sensitized to alpha-hydroxy acids.

Integrating Skin Care Into the Surgical Practice

Anna-Dee Rinehart

The medical profession has begun to recognize the importance of delivering preventive skin-care programs that are cost effective, patient oriented, and able to meet the needs of patients seeking medically sound advice, direction, and emotional support.

The esthetician can provide services for patients to:

- help prevent the outward signs of aging,

- to prevent sun damage,

- to prevent or reduce skin reactions to certain ingredients in products,

- to prevent use of ineffective or harmful skin-care regimens,

- and to prevent and reduce the fear, anxiety, and depression often experienced when considering the options of elective cosmetic procedures.

The plastic surgeon is unable to provide much preventive skin care because of time constraints. The physician can refer patients to the esthetician for an in-depth consultation, developing a plan for continued home care. During the initial consultation the esthetician develops a plan based on the concerns of the patient and the physician's input. The individualized plan is implemented as a part of the overall recommendations resulting from the plastic surgeon's consultation.

An ongoing maintenance program is developed providing skin-care treatments, cosmetic application, education, and resources for the patient to achieve the stated goals, objectives, and outcomes that were defined during the initial consultation. For this part of the esthetician's role in plastic surgery, the esthetician will need to have a well-rounded working knowledge of the services the surgeon offers and why the patient may benefit from these services. It is not the role of the esthetician to recommend that the patient have a cosmetic procedure, but rather to add to the patient's understanding about the options available to achieve the results desired. Men, women, and children desire to have a "normal appearance," to be accepted, to escape the insults of time, trauma, and genetic factors. The integration of estheticians and the implementation of skin care offers patients a chance for high self-esteem, a sense of effectiveness, clarity of choices, courage to face another challenge, and an opportunity to come out of hiding.

Plastic Surgery

The esthetician's role in plastic surgery is two-fold.

1. The esthetician refers patients to the plastic surgeon when the patient's needs exceed cosmetic and skin-care needs.

2. The esthetician works with patients during the preoperative and postoperative phases of elective and reconstructive procedures.

Cosmetic Procedures

A candidate for cosmetic surgery may choose a procedure based on the esthetician's recommendations. For instance, a white female patient seeks the services of the esthetician for a skin-care consultation. During this consultation the esthetician recognizes the redundancy of fat in the jawline, ptosis of the eyelids, or a wide range of other conditions that warrant more than a skin-care treatment. The patient reveals to the esthetician that he or she is concerned about the sagging skin in the neck area and the lines on their face. The esthetician's role is to present the patient with all the options available to deliver the best possible results for the patient's facial concerns. Estheticians need to know when to refer a patient for cosmetic procedures as well as how to handle each procedure before and after.

Preoperative Role of the Esthetician

The esthetician working in a plastic surgeon's office will learn what to look for in patients seeking a facelift or rhytidectomy. The esthetician should be able to conceptualize an image of a so-called "ideal face". This will often give a baseline as to how the "referring role" can best aid the surgeon.

Esthetic Guidelines—Preoperative

1. Assess the patient's cosmetic and skin-care practices.

2. Analyze the skin for quality, texture, and esthetic appearance.

3. Discuss the patient's likes and dislikes in facial appearance.

4. Reassure the patient about the decision for cosmetic surgery.

5. Design a comprehensive skin-care program based on the patient's verbalized needs, the physician's input, and clinical expertise.

6. Educate the patient on preventive measures for diminishing the impact of aging; eighty percent of all outward signs of aging skin are preventable. Tell the patient to:

   Avoid the sun, wind, and extreme weather changes.

   Avoid smoking.

   Avoid/limit fat intake.

   Exercise.

   Eat healthfully.

   Avoid fad diets.

   Use an SPF 15 sunscreen at all times.

   Use moisturizers formulated for their skin type.

7. Teach the patient proper cosmetic application.

8. Promote discussion about the patient's desired outcome for both cosmetic surgery and an ongoing skin-care treatment program.

9. Inform the patient about the limitations and potentials of cosmetic and skin-care products.

10. Gather information about the patient's reasons for having cosmetic surgery.

11. Set goals, plans, and objectives to meet a positive outcome.

12. Teach, inform, direct, and refer the patient to what will be needed to achieve the set goals.

13. Demonstrate to the patient where incisions will be placed, and how to care for them.

14. Give the patient a written home-care guide on postoperative care.

Ideally the patient should see the esthetician at least six weeks before surgery. This allows the esthetician to prepare the patient for healthier skin, discuss the surgery, and answer the patient's concerns as well as educate the patient on ideas of how to wear cosmetics after surgery.

Six Weeks Preoperative

Offer the patient a deep cleansing treatment of the skin. Clean the skin based on assessed needs, using an exfoliant, acne surgery, or moisturizing treatments. Schedule at least one visit to teach the patient about the scars (incision sites) and to demonstrate how cosmetics can conceal those areas. Schedule at least two skin treatments before skin surgery. Inform, direct, and educate the patient at each scheduled visit, addressing the issues of appearance, aging, proper maintenance, scar concealment, cosmetic changes, and specific related surgery issues.

Two Weeks Preoperative

Unfortunately, time may not always permit the patient to utilize the "ideal program". If the patient only has two weeks before their scheduled surgery, it is best to spend one visit teaching and preparing the patient for the surgical procedure and to use the second visit for cosmetic and skin preparation.

Twenty-Four Hours Postoperative

The esthetician may see the facelift patient twenty-four hours postoperatively for the first time. The esthetician's skills in proper cleansing technique and in manipulating the face during the initial postoperative period will be important.

During removal of the bandages the nurse may assist the physician with bandages, scissors, antibiotics, and emotional support of the patient. At times the nurse will not be there for the physician, and the esthetician may have to assist in order to facilitate the patient's care. The physician will remove bandages, check surgical sites, and evaluate the patient's postoperative period.

If the esthetician has the opportunity to work in a hospital setting or a surgical on-site suite, he or she may have a larger role, which may include the following tasks:

1. Once bandages have been removed, the patient is wheeled to the bed of the designated skin-care room.

2. The nurse or assistant will help the patient lie down on the bed.

3. The esthetician will position the patient so that the head is elevated higher than the rest of the body.

4. The wheel chair is removed.

5. Lights in the room should be turned low, especially if the patient's eyes have been done and are sensitive to light.

6. Cover the patient for warmth, as well as because of concerns for modesty and respect.

7. The esthetician should be gloved.

8. The esthetician should position the patient's head on the sink area, in order to wash hair, remove rubber bands, clean the face, apply antibiotics, and reestablish the patient's sense of wellbeing.

9. The esthetician should know the accepted protocol for proper cleansing technique within the medical office or hospital.

10. Once the hair is cleaned, the patient should avoid hair rinses, mousses, hairsprays, or other perfumed, alcohol products.

11. Keep the lights low after cleansing the hair. Assist the patient to the cosmetic area and regown the patient with a clean gown. Assist with the housecoat and shoes. Keep the patient warm.

12. Once the hair is cleansed, recheck the hair for blood and oozing from stitches; observe the amount and intensity of blood and document this information on the patient's chart.

13. Reassure the patient that everything he or she is experiencing is considered normal.

14. Keep the blow dryer a minimum of six to eight inches away from the scalp. Since the surgery is fresh, the patient may feel some numbness and it is easier for the dryer to burn the patient.

15. Do not attempt to do more than simple hair fixing, lipstick, and gentle moisturizer for the facial skin. Keep all products away from wounds!

16. Assist the patient back to the room or ask for help. If the patient is going home, assist the family. Provide the patient with specific, detailed, easy-to-follow instructions for the postoperative care at home. Be sure the patient has topical antibiotics to apply directly to the stitches at home.

As an esthetician within a medical office or hospital, you may or may not be responsible for direct patient care. It is easy to recognize that the role of an esthetician in a plastic surgery practice goes beyond standard protocols as well as esthetic education. The timely contributions of estheticians are innumerable, and they are essential. The physician who works closely with an experienced esthetician will find patients greatly appreciating the program.

One Week to Ten Days Postoperative

The responsible esthetician will have checked on the patient's recovery before the second postoperative period. If possible, you should carry a beeper in order for the patient to reach you. The physician should always be made aware of any contact you and the patient have outside the basic correspondence during the interim of the patient's care. The esthetician is not a physician and should not overstep the boundaries between esthetic management and medical advice. The esthetician's specific role at this time is based on the physician's consent to apply cosmetics and begin skin-care management, which is when the physician actually removes the staples or stitches.

Usually the esthetician begins actively participating in assessment of the wound and deciding if the patient may need more camouflage cosmetics or lymphatic drainage.

The assessment up to this point was done based on the patient's initial consultation, and neither the physician or esthetician can predict the exact results of the surgery or how a patient may feel.

For this reason the postoperative period of any cosmetic surgery should include the following:

The Five R's

1. **REASSESSMENT:** Analyze the skin, observe wounds, note the symmetry of facial features, and compare to initial documentation and pictures. Check the areas of staples and stitches and be sure stitches are not left within suture area.

2. **REDUCE:** Reduce redness, dryness, and flakiness. Each patient is different, and each responds differently to the surgery; each skin type may react with increased dryness, sensitivity, and flakiness due to the trauma of surgery.

3. **REASSURE:** Reassure the patient of their reasons for having the surgery. Remember, cosmetic surgery is an elective surgery and the patient is basically choosing to have the pain and aftereffects to gain an improved/enhanced esthetic appearance. Give the patient support, but do not patronize the patient.

4. **REVIEW:** Review with the patient the need to avoid sun, wind, extreme weather changes, smoking, and alcohol. Remind the patient that the facelift will be beneficial only if he or she makes definite changes toward minimizing the outward effects of aging.

5. **RESCHEDULE:** Reschedule the patient for skin-care treatments. The work began during the six-week pre-op and will continue only if the esthetician encourages the patient.

Four to Six Weeks Postoperative

The patient should be followed up to assure proper management as instructed during the initial consultation and immediate postoperative period. Another important reason the patient should be seen four to six weeks after surgery is to reinforce proper maintenance of the skin. If the patient has chosen not to continue regularly scheduled skin-care visits, this may be the only chance for the esthetician to follow up. At this time the patient may be critical of their results or pleased with the overall surgical experience and esthetic support received. During this visit the esthetician can:

Observe skin quality and texture.

Inspect the patient's own cosmetic application.

Ascertain the patient's receptiveness to continuing in the skin-care program.

Document whether the program was able to achieve the goals set at the initial consultation.

Evaluate the objectives set with the patient and allow the patient to agree or disagree with the outcome.

Confirm the patient's feelings about the results of the surgery and how, if any, the skin-care program helped in acceptance of the cosmetic decision and results.

Use the Five R's.

While this may be the final visit for some patients, others will eagerly embrace ongoing skin-care treatments.

The esthetician's role may vary depending on the type of surgical procedure performed. Blepharoplasties, upper and lower lid resections, require special attention post-operatively from the esthetician.

Eyelid Surgery—Postoperative Twenty-Four Hours

Begin to inspect the incision sites prior to any cleaning.

Observe for infection, hematomas, or stitches left accidentally.

Never apply pressure to "fix" appearance of eyes.

Clean eye area with cool water compresses to remove the residue of blood and serous fluid.

Start cleaning movements from the inner canthus to the outer, with gentle light stroking.

Repeat this movement with another swab, and never use cotton when cleaning a wound.

Apply a swab saturated with water and hydrogen peroxide directly to the incisions.

Clean each eye separately with a swab, and do not cross-clean both eyes.

Apply topical antibiotic with a swab in one direction, and use one swab on each eye. (This is sometimes done by a nurse, but as the physician recognizes how to use the esthetician in patient care, it will be helpful for you to learn as much as possible.)

Once finished cleaning an eye, use cool compresses to soothe the eye and reduce swelling.

Keep the head elevated and do not pull, stretch, or strain the patient's facial features.

Give the patient and family member postoperative instructions for home care.

Be sure the patient can reach you for any cosmetic or esthetic concern.

Eyelid Surgery—Postoperative Seven to Ten Days

During this visit the stitches are removed. If there is no evidence of a hematoma, and no signs or symptoms of infection (heat, redness, swelling), you can begin to execute the plan set in the initial consultation.

Common Concerns About Eyelid Surgery

The patient may express concern about uneven eye appearance. He or she may state that they look uneven. Still others may feel the physician left one eye with an excess of skin. These are typical concerns. You should allow the patient to vent these concerns and assure the patient that the healing process will change the appearance of the eyes. Instruct and demonstrate for the patient how to apply ointment to the eye skin, gently using a rolling method. This rolling technique minimizes pressure on the delicate eye area.

Six Weeks Postoperative for Eyelid Surgery

1. Apply the principles of reevaluation at each visit.

2. Measure the eye distance; share and explore different eye techniques.

3. Use camouflage techniques, but try to discourage the patient from using thick makeup.

4. Take another photo so that the patient may compare/contrast the before and after.

5. Support the patient, but do not disregard the patient's concerns about their appearance.

6. Have materials available for the patient to learn new eye-makeup techniques.

7. Samples of cosmetics are helpful.

Cosmetics and Camouflage Therapy

The surgeon has long recognized the importance of cosmetics and the role they play in the patient's recovery. These basic guidelines were established by estheticians who have worked directly with burn survivors and surgical patients.

1. Select one foundation that is a shade lighter and another a shade darker than the patient's skin. Apply one part light and one part dark and mix until you have achieved a natural-looking foundation.

2. If the skin is oilier than normal, a translucent powder will dry the small amount of oil present. If the patient must use powder, use it sparingly.

3. To reduce redness, use a green cover stick. Apply it with a cosmetic sponge. Apply gently but firmly to the entire face. The green will neutralize the redness, and the foundation will go on smoothly.

4. Use any color on the eyes except red, fuchsia, and pink. These colors will bring back out the redness under the foundation that needs to be neutralized.

5. Eyeliner colors should be chosen according to taste first, then hair color, the time of day, the clothes, and where the patient will be going.

6. Cheek color can be chosen based on what has already been done. Stay away from pink undertones. Warm colors may have an orange tone when applied to a healing face. Choose a color with sand or brown undertones.

7. Do not use any frosted or iridescent colors on the lips, eyes, or cheeks. They only accent fine lines and wrinkles.

8. The matte look has a more natural appearance than any other cosmetic application.

9. For short hair, and a really different look, try hairpieces and wigs.

10. Try to experiment a bit more, and do not stick to the same makeup application, hairdo, or wardrobe.

Contraindications for Cosmetic Use

1. Bleeding at incision site.

2. Signs and symptoms of infection: heat, redness, swelling.

3. Patient verbalizes dislike of cosmetics.

4. Known sensitivities, allergic reactions.

5. Open sores or wounds.

❡ Review and Summary ❡

The various types of esthetic treatments that could be offered in a medical practice have been discussed. However, I reemphasize that there must be a consultation between the physician and the esthetician to determine what treatments will actually benefit the patient. Ultimately the physician will choose what treatments will be of medical or scientific value to the patient. What do I mean by that? If you want to perform a treatment on acneic skin that includes having the patient stand on his or her head for five minutes, then you must have the scientific data to back up that treatment plan. Remember, most physicians do not know what is involved in an esthetic treatment or know what level of training you received in esthetic school.

Scientific data was presented in this chapter regarding lymphatic drainage and its use in the pre- and postoperative patient to help reduce ecchymosis and erythema. The esthetician and the physician can now intelligently discuss the benefits of adding this service to available treatments. The types of ingredients used in facial masks have proven chemical properties that help to reduce (*p. acnes*) bacteria and assist in reducing TEWL (*trans epidermal water loss*).

Identifying wounds and having knowledge of the skin's restoration process can go a long way in convincing the physician that adding esthetic treatments to his/her practice will in fact play an integral role in the care of the postoperative patient. If the opportunity arises to work in a burn unit with burn survivors, the esthetician's expertise in complications that may occur, including loss of sweat and sebaceous glands, will help in understanding the patient's concerns.

Chemical agents and their use is presented conservatively in this chapter, however, to validate their serious nature. An esthetician must be proficient in obtaining complete patient histories. The treatment of acne patients has always been a stronghold for the esthetician in the medical practice, and the presentation of this acne study can help reinforce the effectiveness of this treatment.

The role of the esthetician in the surgical setting was explored through preoperative assessment, development of a treatment plan, and follow-through postoperatively.

Many opportunities will be available in the medical arena, and the esthetician who chooses to read and become educated will excel in this promising new career field. Good luck!

References

[1]C. Clayman, "Lymphatic System", *Journal American Medical Association* 12 (1989):656.

[2]H. Wittlinger, G. Wittlinger, *Textbook of Dr. Vodder's Manual Lymph Drainage*, Vol 1, translated by Harris R. Haug International, Brussels.

[3]R. Harris, "An Introduction to Manual Lymph Drainage—The Vodder Method", *Massage Therapy Journal* (1992):55–66.

[4]P. Pugliese, L. Garofallou, "Lymphatic Drainage Massage", in *Principles and Practices of Opthalmic Plastic and Reconstructive Surgery I & II*, Stephen Bosniak, M.D., Ed. (W.B. Saunders Company, 1995):651–656.

[5]P.O. Hutzschenreuter, H. Wittlinger, G. Wittlinger, I. Kurtz, "Post-Mastectomy Arm Lymph Edema: Treated by Manual Lymph Drainage and Compression Bandage Therapy", *European Journal of Physical Medicine and Rehabilitation 1* (1991): 166–170.

[6]P.D. Mc Master, "Conditions in the Skin Influencing Interstitial Fluid Movement, Lymph Formation and Lymph Flow", *Annals New York Academy of Sciences* 46 (1976):743."

[7]J. Daroczy, "Manner of Function", in *The Dermal Lymphatic Capillaries,* (Berlin: Springer-Verlag, 1988) 81–83; G. Wang, S. Zhong, "Experimental Study of Lymphatic Contractility and its Clinical Importance", *Annals of Plastic Surgery* 15 (1995):284; J.G. Hall, B. Morris, G. Wooley, "Intrinsic Rhythmic Propulsion of Lymph in the Sheep", *Journal of Physiology* 180 (1965):336–348.

[8]Reprinted with permission, J. Naughton, T. Zimmerman: Burn Care, *PCI Journal of Progressive Clinical Insights* 3,5 (1995): 11.

[9]Burn Rehabilitation, National Institute for Burn Medicine, 6,5 (1983) 3–4.

[10]Reprinted with permission, Esthetics, Manufacturers and Distributors Alliance. (1996)

[11]A.R. Shalita, P.E. Pochi, J.J. Leyden, "Acne Therapy in the 90s", *Postgrad Med 4* (1991): 3–15.

[12]N.S. Sadick, "Therapeutic Skin Treatments found Important in Cystic Inflammatory Acne", *Cos Derm* 6, 9(1993): 29–34.

Chapter Three

Charting
Your Course

In this chapter you will learn:

- the initial steps you need to take if this is what you've decided is the right career move for you

- the importance of planning your career

- how to put that plan into action

- how to create a job description

- how to put together a resumé

- how to write a cover letter

Embarking on a career or changing the direction of the work you're already doing can be frightening at first because the distance between where you are and where you want to be—or where you think you want to be—can seem so vast. The first step on any journey into the unknown is always the most difficult, and the good news is that you're actually on your way. The very fact that you're reading this book means that you've already taken the first step toward defining a successful career—you're exploring your options.

Planning—The Basis
of a Successful Career

You'd be amazed at how many people never bother to plan their careers. They plan just about everything else about their lives—

vacations, weddings, even grocery shopping—but when it comes to what they spend most of their working lives doing, they drift. Most people never actually examine where they want to go; they simply follow the crowd and do the obvious. But even if what you eventually wind up doing is the more obvious and usual choice—for estheticians that would be working in a salon—it won't really be your choice unless you actively, consciously make it. I don't think working in a medical setting is the right choice for every esthetician, nor do I think that every esthetician working in a medical practice should do it to the exclusion of other esthetic work. I know it's the right choice for me because I made it only after spending a great deal of time thinking about what I like, what I'm good at, and what my options are, given my predilections and my training.

And that's really the key for any important career decision. It's a cliché, but it's true; if you like what you do, you're much more likely to be successful at it. But really knowing what you like is not as easy as it might seem. Many of us took tests in high school to find out what we were best suited for. Those tests, among other things, were really subtle explorations of what we enjoyed doing. A number of books out there describe exercises you can do to uncover what you really enjoy, and if you've never taken the time to do this kind of thing, I suggest you try it. A classic in the field is the paperback *What Color is Your Parachute*, by Richard N. Bolles (published by Ten Speed Press in Berkeley, California).

Even if you don't have much faith in the specific techniques these books employ, doing the exercises at least forces you to think about the direction you'd like to take, as opposed to what you think you ought to be doing with your life. Whatever exercises you use, they should have one thing in common: they should help you free your mind from the strictures we usually place on it when we think about work. In other words, when you think about what you'd like to be doing with your career, you shouldn't be limited to what you traditionally think of as work. The whole point of these exercises, in fact, is to broaden your usual definitions of work. Think of the things you actually choose to do when you're completely free to spend your time as you like. That includes what you do for entertainment, volunteer activities, hobbies, even cleaning the garage if that gives you pleasure. In fact, the things you wouldn't think of under ordinary circumstances can be most revealing. If you like cleaning the garage (and people like to do much stranger things, after all) it may mean you enjoy bringing order out of chaos.

Other exercises are useful for helping define what shape you'd like your career to take. Priority lists, where you list the pros and cons of a decision on each side of a piece of paper and give numerical weights to each entry to see which side comes out ahead, decision trees, or any of a host of methods used to clarify decisions can be used. Make lists of goals for your next position—wealth, challenge, interaction with interesting people, creativity, a pleasant environment, adventure, fame, power, leadership opportunities, long lunch hours, anything you want—and try to imagine the ideal position. Pay attention to what excites you and what doesn't.

Remember, these exercises are for your benefit. Be as free as you can, because their only purpose is to help you think creatively about your strengths and to become conscious of the forces that help you succeed or prevent you from doing as well as you can.

No one should make important decisions without serious consideration. But for the esthetician, it's especially important to articulate what we want because no one has really done it for us. This is a new field, and definitions of what it involves have not yet been developed. That's not to say there is no information about estheticians working with physicians, but it's more likely to be available in professional journals than in books, and it's not yet a topic covered in all schools. In a sense, those of us who choose to work in a medical setting are defining the field of "clinical" esthetics. And that means we're going to have to explain what we do, or what we want to do, to people who have very little idea about it, including the physicians we will be working with. If we're not clear about what a esthetician does in a medical setting, they certainly won't be. This brings us to the next section, formulating a job description.

Formulating a Job Description

How do you write a **job description** for a job that doesn't have hard and fast outlines? Actually, it's not as difficult as it at first seems. From the first and second chapters, which reviewed the options available, you should have a broad idea about what estheticians can do in a medical setting. Now more details should be added. The purpose of doing this is three-fold: first, it will clarify the job for yourself; second, it will help you communicate it to others; and finally, you'll use it as the basis for cover letters to physicians.

What we're talking about here is not the kind of job description that human resources departments expect to receive. It's not a detailed list of your duties and responsibilities as much as an outline of the role you'll play in a physician's office. As such, it will cover three basic areas: the direct work you'll do with patients, your role as a marketing person, and the administrative work you'll do. This is not an hour-by-hour description of your working day. Rather, it's a blueprint of the new capabilities you'll be bringing to the physician's practice. As such, it can work as a marketing tool to help "sell" a physician on the idea of hiring you to perform certain work that will enhance the services he/she can offer patients and increase the overall profitability of the practice.

Patient Services

This section of the job proposal outlines the kinds of services you'll perform for patients, including both the treatments you'll offer and the education you'll help provide. Don't be exhaustive. Each physician's practice is organized differently, and while some physicians may want you to perform certain procedures, others may not. Regardless of the type of practice (i.e., dermatology, plastic, or reconstructive, etc.), you can describe certain procedures and practices that you can safely assume will be required.

Patient Evaluation and Education

As an expert in cosmetics and skin care, you can assume that you'll play an important role in evaluating patients on their first visit and in educating them on the role of cosmetics and the proper skin care techniques. Specifically, an esthetician in a surgical practice will typically advise the patient in the weeks before surgery about what cosmetics to avoid, how to keep the skin clean, and how to make sure the skin and underlying tissues are in the best possible condition. The physician may also delegate to the esthetician responsibility for educating the patient about the role of nutrition and hydration prior to surgery.

In a dermatology practice, the esthetician may be responsible for obtaining the patient's history, including a complete list of the products the patient uses, any history of allergy or contact dermatitis associated with any of them, as well as a description of the techniques the patient uses to clean and maintain the skin. Because estheticians are generally much more knowledgeable about cosmetic products than physicians, the esthetician is particularly well qualified to question the patient about their use. The history should also include information about what salon services the patient has had and any reaction that might have occurred as a result. Of particular importance is the history of chemical exfoliations, past cosmetic surgeries, and any topical and/or oral medications being used.

Obtaining a history is important for several reasons. It may, of course, have a direct bearing on the subsequent medical diagnosis or evaluation, and it gives both the physician and the esthetician the background they need to set the best course for the patient subsequent to the specific medical treatment or surgical procedure. It also saves the physician a great deal of time, which can then be devoted directly to patient care. And the esthetician can ask questions and uncover information that the patient might not think relevant, but that may in fact be quite important. In a dermatologic setting the esthetician's role is to help the patient understand the pathogenesis (causes) of acne and educate the patient about what factors, such as products containing oil and sun exposure, will worsen or exacerbate their condition. It is also to assist the patient regarding cleansing treatments, which would include exfoliation and acne surgery (removal of comedones, milia, etc.) which will help to prevent acne from increasing or flaring again.

The Psychological Advantage

Estheticians bring another important advantage to this aspect of patient care—a psychological advantage. Patients are often more comfortable talking to an esthetician about their cosmetic concerns than they are talking to a physician about them. The esthetician is less intimidating, and the patient knows that the esthetician will treat these concerns with respect. The role of educator continues throughout the patient's treatment. The esthetician will continually review how the patient is complying with the medical procedure, answer any questions, and make sure the patient understands how to properly follow any home care instructions the physician has prescribed. Postsurgically, the patient will have to learn new ways to clean the skin, and it will be largely the responsibility of the esthetician to instruct the patient. The esthetician will also make sure the patient understands any special instructions the physician may have given about diet and physical activity, including the importance of avoiding sun exposure. Some patients will present special challenges, especially children, the elderly, and those with disabilities. The esthetician should receive special training, either from the physician or in special courses taught at professional meetings, that the physician suggests (and pays for) if your responsibilities include handling these special situations.

Home-Care Instruction

For cosmetic and reconstructive surgical patients, home-care instruction is particularly important. Here again, you aren't expected to know how to handle these situations without further training, but estheticians in surgical practices can expect to spend a fair amount of time helping patients understand the special precautions they need to take during the period of healing following the procedure. Patients who have had rhinoplasty, for instance, or any of the procedures involved with facial cosmetic surgery, will need to learn special techniques for cleansing the skin during the time when the new tissue is still unstable. The esthetician may also suggest or provide special non-oily lotions to be used during this period and provide special camouflage cosmetics and techniques to minimize the effects of bruising (**ecchymosis**) and redness (**erythema**).

Finally, and perhaps most important, especially for the surgery patient, the esthetician will design new makeup for the patient to take advantage of the work the surgeon has done to remodel the face. Cosmetic techniques the patient had used to compensate for the defects that have been corrected will no longer be appropriate, and new ways to apply makeup can very significantly enhance the work the surgeon has done. In many ways, this can be the most rewarding part of working in a medical setting, because your special expertise can make the difference between a mere improvement and a really spectacular change in the patient's appearance. It's one thing to give a client a makeover in a salon; it's quite another to help a patient

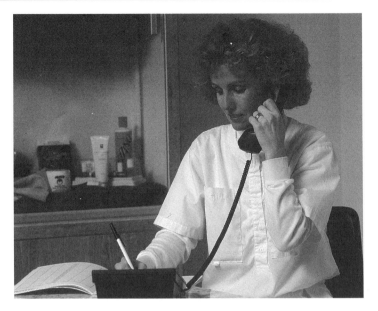

Emphasize that you intend to become a full-fledged member of the practice team.

fully realize the transformation that can occur following surgery.

Administrative Responsibilities

Although it will be the most rewarding part of your day, not all of your time will be spent with patients. You'll also undertake a certain number of administrative responsibilities, although precisely what these will be will depend on the nature and size of the practice you join. Larger practices may well have a practice administrator in place, and she or he may take on some of the duties you would perform in a smaller practice. Whatever the size of the practice you hope to join, however, your purpose in approaching the physician for the first time should be to emphasize the added value you'll bring to his or her practice; that value will be diminished if, by adding your esthetic services, the physician increases the work of an already overworked staff. To minimize the burdens on the physician's staff, which in many practices is limited to a receptionist and/or a nurse, you should detail the administrative tasks you are prepared to undertake.

These administrative duties can be divided into areas: general practice administration and administrative tasks related specif-

ically to esthetic functions. We'll consider each later, particularly
in Chapter Seven, "Practice Administration". Two points need to
be made here, however. Emphasize that you intend to become a
full-fledged member of the practice team. That means you are
willing to learn the practice's administrative procedures and help
out when necessary in such routine functions as scheduling,
answering phones, and perhaps filling in for the receptionist on
occasion. And you should make it clear that you are prepared to
handle all of the administrative chores that relate solely to your
services. Of course, some of these will have to be coordinated
with the rest of the staff—scheduling and documentation, for
instance—but you should assume responsibility for those chores
that relate specifically to your role in the practice, such as ordering your own supplies (professional and retail) and displaying
educational material that deals specifically with your services.

The point is, if you want to maximize the advantages of hiring you, you have to minimize the disadvantages, and increased
administrative burdens, especially in this time of burgeoning
demands on practices from insurance companies and government regulators, should be avoided. If you take on the responsibility for any additional administrative tasks hiring you entails,
you effectively answer the objection that the practice can't
accommodate increased administrative overhead.

One word of caution: don't overdo it; don't offer more than
you're willing to do. It's one thing to be responsible for the
administration of the new elements you bring to the physician's
practice and quite another to volunteer to become a part-time
office administrator. If you wanted to spend most of your time as
a medical receptionist, you wouldn't be reading this book.

Putting Together a Targeted Resumé

The job description is designed to clarify, both for you and
for the physician, just what you'll be adding to the physician's
practice. It can be a great marketing tool, but it's just one part of
the package. The other essential document is your resumé.

We've all heard the clichés about resumés: they're just
excuses not to interview someone; if you want yours to be
noticed, print it on chartreuse paper; keep it brief; make it long;
include a picture; don't include a picture; type it in red ink on

Paige Katherine Wooldridge
111 South Street
Springs, New York 22222
Tel (111) 555-2121

EDUCATION

1978	High School Graduation Diploma, Forest Hill Collegiate, Toronto.
1979–1980	Makeup Artistry Diploma, International Top Models, Toronto.
Sept 1988– Feb 1989	Completed six-month diploma course in esthetics. Edith Serei School, Toronto.
May 1990	Completed two-month Advanced Esthetic Course, which included nutrition, manual lymphatic drainage, body treatments. Edith Serei School, Toronto.
Jan 1992– Mar 1992	Trained with a leading dermatologist to further advance my knowledge of skin diseases and disorders and their medical treatment, Toronto.

TRAINING SEMINARS ATTENDED

Feb 1994	Seminar in theory and practice in paramedical camouflage. Specialized training in the Glyderm procedure, doing glycolic peels and product knowledge of the Glyderm line.
June 1994	Training in the Systeme Avance skin and body care treatments.
Feb 1990	Rene Guinot advanced training seminar. Makeup seminar with Mac Cosmetics (Photography and runway makeup).
Aug 1989	Aromatherapy course with Patricia Miller.
Sept 1987	Training in Facial and Body Therapy with Ann Gallant.

PRACTICAL EXPERIENCE

Aug 1993– Present	Kirsch Camouflage Clinic Duties include: facials, face peels, waxing, makeup, camouflage.
June 1994– Present	The Institute of Cosmetic Surgery, Dr. Lorne Tarshis Duties include: Glycolic exfoliations, facials, makeup, camouflage for patients after cosmetic surgery, skin care consultation.
Sept 1992– Aug 1993	Zehava School of Esthetics Duties included: Assisting in teaching the full-time esthetic course to students.
June 1991– Oct 1991	Phytoderm Inc. Duties included: Sales consultant promoting a new skin-care line from France. Laid off due to market conditions.
July 1990– June 1991	Edith Serei Esthetic School Duties included: Full-time teaching of esthetic course to students and part-time work in the salon.
Sept 1989– June 1990	Esthetics of Paige Duties included: Full-time esthetician.
Feb 1989– July 1989	Patricia Miller Esthetic Skincare Duties included: Part-time esthetician.
July 1987– Aug 1988	Operated a small esthetic business in Toronto.

VOLUNTEER WORK

Sept 1993– Present	"Look Good, Feel Better" program to help women cancer patients improve their appearance and self-image by teaching them hands-on beauty techniques.

the back of a hundred dollar bill. Forget the clichés. There's no getting around the fact that you need a resumé, but in my experience, you need a particular kind of resumé, and you don't have to worry about yours getting lost in the crowd. At the moment there is no crowd. Your resumé won't be used to narrow a large field of applicants; rather, it will serve to reinforce the impression you make on the physician with your initial approach, and it will quickly document your experience and your expertise.

What kind of resumé works best? In this case, I recommend a targeted resumé. This contradicts the advice given by the majority of books about resumés. For most purposes, the chronological resumé works best because it's easier to organize and easier for the person screening applicants to read. For our purposes, however, the chronological resumé is usually pointless, unless you have extensive prior experience working in physicians' offices. What's more, while your salon experience, other work experience, and your education are all important, the physician you hope to work with will be most interested in what skills and experience you have that can be directly related to the work you'll perform in a medical office.

The **targeted resumé** is highly focused and directed to a specific job target. It is less a history of what you've already done than a clear presentation of the skills you'll need to perform a specific job in the future. For that reason, it's particularly useful in a new and growing field such as esthetics; for most of us, working in a physician's practice is a departure from our past work experience, so it's unlikely there will be other jobs in your history that exactly match the one you're applying for now. For that matter, it's very unlikely the physician to whom you're applying ever hired someone like you. It's a new role for which the physician has no exact points of comparison. The resumé, then, like the job description we've been talking about, will help to define the job while at the same time presenting you as the ideal person to fill it.

The targeted resumé I'm suggesting should begin with a statement that summarizes the strengths you'll bring to the practice. You know what those are, but they should probably include your expertise in esthetics, your experience working with a broad range of clients, your ability to sell and cross-sell services, and your management and administrative skills. Although your experience in salons—your own or working for someone else—will

Philip Baker
200 Long Road
N. Beach, California
(555) 212-1001

EXPERIENCE

1993 to Present   **ESTHETICIAN**
Esties' International

Services Offered

- Facials
- Extractions
- Neck Massage
- Waxing
- Lash & Brow Tinting
- Manual Massage
- Back Massage
- Glycolic Peels
- Artificial Lashes &Brows
- Cellulite Body Treatments
- Make-up: Day & Evening, Special Effects, Ramp, Paramedical Camouflage

MACHINE EXPERIENCE

- Sorisa Belex 04 (galvanic, toning, firming)
- Bio-Derm GT7000 (galvanic, toning, firming)
- Bio Therapeutic Computer (microcurrent)
- Time Machine (hand-held galvanic)
- Rita McQueen (infared/massage)

AWARDS/CERTIFICATIONS

- Advanced Peeling Techniques & Marketing Strategies
- Acne, Ethnic Skin & Pigmentation Disorders
- Special Effects Make-up Workshop I
- Special Effects Make-up Workshop II
- Images of Success Paramedical Camouflage Make-up
- Bio-Derm Certificate
- Certificate of Appreciation, Cancer Society
- MD Formulations, Peel Techniques

EDUCATION

- Je Boutique Beauty Cosmetology
- 400 Additional Hours—Esthetician
- Glycolic Treatments (Additional information is available upon request.)
- Make-up Classes (Additional information is available upon request.)

SPECIAL SERVICES

- American Cancer Society ("Look Good, Feel Better")
- Make-up Instructor

REFERENCES   Available upon request.

probably be where you nurtured most of these skills, don't limit yourself to salon experience. Draw on your entire work history, volunteer activities, academic record, and hobbies.

How the Resumé Should be Structured

I need hardly tell you that appearance counts, but I'm not going to get specific about what typefaces you should use or exactly how to arrange your resumé; there are enough books readily available to help you with the mechanical details and to provide samples you can follow. The content too can be flexible, but you should start with a general statement that summarizes your strengths. Here's an example:

> Over five years experience in every aspect of esthetics in a salon setting. Comprehensive experience managing skin-care programs for a wide variety of clients, with special emphasis on problematic skin. Extraction of comedones and milia; hydration of the skin; the proper use of cosmetics to enhance appearance; and the use of cosmetics to camouflage defects in skin structure and color. Experience in the removal of unwanted facial and body hair, including waxing and electrolysis. Successful track record selling high-end line of skin-care products to salon clients. Management of inventory including ordering and inventory control. Additional training in psychology with a minor in biology at XYZ University.

Obviously, if you've had specific medical experience, put that up front, including any work you've done with physicians and any specific medical training you've had. Include courses you've taken in ancillary fields, such as psychology or counseling, and if you've had real experience working with a particular group, such as teenagers or the elderly, mention that.

The summary statement is meant to be broad; this is the place to boast. You don't have to document anything here or back it up with specifics; that comes later, but remember that anything you say in this opening statement should be expanded on in the body of the resumé. If you've handled ordering supplies and selling cosmetics, mention that here and get specific about it later.

Next comes a list of your specific skills, beginning with skin care and applied esthetics—if at all possible, these should be two separate entries, since they are of primary importance to the physician considering hiring you. Here's where you should be specific. Under skin care, for instance, mention the procedures you've done and the number and variety of skin types that you've worked with. This should be a comprehensive entry that not only lists the kinds of services you've provided, such as deep cleansing and hydrating facials, chemical exfoliations, etc., but also the methods and the equipment you've used. If you've treated particularly challenging cases, mention them and the success you've had with them. In particular, detail any experience you've had in which patients who came to you with chronic problems, such as acne, have improved and been able to maintain healthier skin.

If you have experience in electrolysis, make that a separate heading. Dermatologists, in particular, frequently treat patients for conditions that result in unwanted hair, and treatment with electrolysis is often used along with treatment of the underlying medical condition.

Expand your list of skills, using a separate heading for each one, until you've covered everything you think might be relevant. If you've had experience helping trauma or burn survivors using camouflage techniques, highlight it. If you've dealt with clients with special psychological needs, that's another special skill you'll want to give prominence to. One way to make sure you haven't short-changed yourself in describing your skills is to think of the patients who are likely to present themselves to the kind of medical specialty you want to work with and ask yourself if you've had clients like them.

This leads me to a word of caution. You're not a physician, and you'll quickly alienate potential physician-employers if you try to present yourself as a medical expert or, worse still, someone who actually "treats" medical conditions without a medical license. In fact, this is a sensitive area in certain cases, especially when patients have acne, other skin lesions, or photo-damaged skin that may be the result, at least in part, of poor skin care, the use of the wrong cosmetics, and failure to use sun blocks. Since one of the important benefits of using the services of a skilled esthetician is healthier skin, you can be expected to advise patients on these matters, advice that will in many cases be identical to the advice a physician would offer. But you'll alienate physicians if you present yourself as duplicating their services.

Remember that you have special expertise, especially in the use of skin-care products, and you have broad experience in helping patients move from careless or unhealthy skin-care practices to techniques designed to establish better conditions.

Once you've described your special skills, you might add a section on related experience, if you've had any. This is particularly important if you've worked in any medical or medically related fields; naturally, if you're a nurse or have had medical assisting experience, you'll list it here; obviously, that kind of information would have been included in your summary statement, but here is where you would go into further detail.

What other related experience warrants inclusion? Pharmacy work, any kind of counseling work, work as a health aide, and any experience you've had, including volunteer experience, in any medically related field. If you're a volunteer with your local ambulance unit, that's relevant. Don't go too far afield, however. A reputation as the makeup expert when you worked as a receptionist is hardly a professional qualification, although your experience as a receptionist might be of interest to a prospective employer. Extensive experience doing makeup for a local theater group is something you might include, although you can definitely skip experience as a volunteer face-painter at the local county fair. What to include and what to leave out is a judgment call, but don't include things just to fill up space; irrelevant entries detract from your genuine skills, and they're also a waste of the physician's time.

After your skills, you should list your employment history. This should be a chronological listing, and it should leave no gaps unexplained. Don't go into detail about each job; simply list the dates, your position, and the company you worked for. If you dropped out of the workforce for any reason, explain it. And don't worry if some of these jobs are unrelated to your work as an esthetician; in the targeted resumé, the job history is much less important than it is in the traditional chronological resumé.

The next section, your educational history, is important. Here's where you'll list your education since high school, in chronological order, including the institution you attended, the degrees or certificates you earned, and the fields you concentrated in. This list should include not only the standard academic programs, but any professional programs you've completed, including special training offered by cosmetic or pharmaceutical companies. And don't forget professional seminars and conferences you've attended. Make sure you include any formal training you've had in medically related areas, such as training in first aid, CPR, and volunteering in an ambulance unit. If your degree is not in one of the sciences, you might mention specific courses you've taken, like a medical terminology class, especially if it was more advanced than the basic courses for non-science majors. Once again, the rule is to include everything that helps demonstrate how you will work well in a medical practice and how you will broaden the benefits of that practice to its patients.

Finally, include a section on awards you've won, articles you've published, and any professional affiliations you maintain, particularly membership in esthetic organizations.

Writing Your Cover Letter

If you've come this far, if you've planned your campaign, put together a meaningful job description, and written an effective, targeted resumé, you've invested a considerable amount of time and effort in what you intend to be a new and rewarding career practicing esthetics in a medical setting.

Perhaps the single most common mistake job seekers make is to spend a great deal of time and effort creating the perfect resumé and then investing five minutes in the cover letter that will convey it to a prospective employer. I can understand why people make that mistake, but I strongly urge you not to. Cover letters, unlike resumés, even targeted resumés, must be written specifically for each prospective employer. They take time to write, and even people who are comfortable with writing about specific topics often find it difficult to write this kind of letter, which is usually directed to a stranger but which should convey something of your personality as well as your strengths in a somewhat personal way. Fortunately, you needn't rely entirely on creative inspiration; there are definite rules to follow that can guide you in creating an effective cover letter.

At best, your cover letter will convey a strong impression of who and what you are and stimulate so much interest in you that the reader will decide to interview you even before he or she has read your resumé. At the very least, your letter should do nothing to detract from the impression your resumé is designed

Sample Cover Letter to Physician

Dear Dr.:

I'd like to take this opportunity to introduce myself to you. I am a licensed esthetician in the State of New York, and I am presently working in a full-service salon, which offers hair, nail and skin-care services.

As an esthetician I perform a variety of skin-care services that help to enhance a client's skin by exfoliation of dead skin cells, cleansing and extraction of comedones, and hydration of the skin. I also have the ability to assist facial-surgery clients in returning to their normal routines by the application of camouflage cosmetics, which cover bruising and redness.

I have gained much experience over the last three years working in a salon; however, I feel that I can best utilize my talents in a medical setting. If you have not already thought about setting up esthetic skin-care services in your practice, I would very much like the opportunity to meet with you and discuss the benefits for you and your patients.

I will call you in two weeks, after you have had a chance to review my resumé, and see when you would like to meet with me. Thank you in advance for your consideration.

Sincerely,

Your name, typed

Enclosure—Resume

to create. At worst, a sloppy, poorly written cover letter can actually serve to irrevocably drive any thought of meeting you from the physician's mind.

The Absolute Minimum

First, let's make sure the basics are covered. Your cover letter is analogous to a book cover; its purpose is to entice the reader to look further, first to your resumé and then to a personal interview. And since it's the first contact the physician has with you, it conveys the all-important first impression, and first impressions are hard to dislodge. If it's positive, it's likely you'll get an interview; if it's negative, your chances are very slim, regardless of how impressive your resumé is.

At the very least, the cover letter must be attractive, free of spelling and grammatical errors, and personally addressed to the physician, using the full name he or she prefers for professional purposes. You should use a standard business format, either indented or block (if you're not familiar with how business letters look, check any of the many books on writing business letters readily available at any library). Don't fax your letter; mail it. Use white or cream paper.

What should you say? Basically, you should cover four points:

1. The purpose of the letter.

2. Why you want to become a member of the physician's team.

3. What you will contribute to it.

4. When and how you intend to follow up to schedule an interview.

Each of these elements, except the third, should be tailored to your specific target. Your opening paragraph—it can be a single sentence in some cases—explains why you're writing. That sounds simplistic, but it's important to present yourself as decisive and efficient from the start, and this is a good way to do it. If you're writing cold, without an introduction or referral, simply state that you're writing because you want to explore the possibility of joining the physician's practice as a specialist in esthetics. If you've been referred by a third person, say that you're writing at the suggestion of *X*, who thought physician *Y* would be interested in augmenting his practice with an esthetician. If you've previously met the physician, say so and continue with your purpose.

If at all possible, your next paragraph should demonstrate some knowledge of the practice you want to join. That will require some research, but it's well worth putting in time at the library in order to demonstrate your knowledge of the specialty in general and of the physician you're writing to in particular. Perhaps the physician has been quoted in the press, written articles in magazines or newspapers, or appeared on local television or radio shows. Mention that you're familiar with what he or she has said, and, if at all possible, relate it to your expertise in esthetics. If the physician has written anything about cosmetics, for instance, you can turn that into a perfect opening to sell your services to the practice. If there's been anything in the press about the physician that relates to one of your special interests, such as helping children with congenital deformities, use that as a starting point.

If you haven't been able to uncover anything about the practice in the press, you'll have to be general in your approach, but the more specific, the better. Definitely look at recent issues of the professional journals in the practice's specialty, and don't neglect the more general medical journals, such as the *PCI Journal of Progressive Clinical Insights* or *Cosmetic Dermatology* (see the Appendix for a complete list of journals).

The next paragraph should describe what you can bring to the practice. Remember, this isn't your resumé, it's an introduction to your resumé, so keep it brief. That's actually harder than it sounds because you only have a few sentences to convey the essence of your skills, but if you've written a good job description and if you've paid attention to the skills section in your targeted resumé, this paragraph shouldn't be too much of a challenge. And the good thing is, you can probably use it in any cover letter you write. One technique that helps in making this paragraph both concise and effective is to concentrate on results, not responsibilities, and be as specific as possible, especially about anything that can be quantified. If you've boosted the client base at a salon, for instance, say by how much. If you've increased product sales, say by what percent. But this needn't be just a numbers exercise. This is the paragraph where you'll talk about yourself, so put it in personal terms. If you've had a success with a client you're particularly proud of, mention it and say how that's the kind of work you look forward to doing in the physician's practice.

Your conclusion should be a statement about how and when you'll contact the office to arrange an interview. Don't be shy. Some people avoid saying they'll call to set up an appointment because they think it's too aggressive. On the contrary! It shows initiative and actually relieves the physician of the need to take the next step. Don't worry; if he or she doesn't want to see you, you won't get the appointment. But too many good opportunities are lost because applicants rely on busy physicians to take the time and effort to contact them. By writing, you've already taken the first step; follow through by saying you'll call in a week or two to see if an appointment would be mutually worthwhile.

❦ Review and Summary ❦

Only in the last few years has the career option of working in a medical practice become available. Without proper education, it is difficult and maybe frightening at first to decide whether working in a medical practice is for you. Additional training is needed and at this time there is very little support from state schools in offering medical education. You need to determine if this type of position is for you. It will be challenging; you will interact with people who may have facial anomalies or other concerns over their appearance, so you must show patience and understanding and at all times be conscious of the patient's confidentiality in regard to their treatment.

Formulating a job description for an area that is this new and is certainly not well defined can seem a little overwhelming. The job description of an esthetician in a medical practice can vary widely, depending on the physician's philosophy of what an esthetician can do in the practice, and how the physician views the role of the esthetician versus the other health-care providers, such as the nurse or physician's assistant. Patient evaluation and education in the area of cosmetics and the general health of the skin will be an important role for the esthetician.

A psychological advantage is that an esthetician spends an entire hour with the patient; a lot of information may be gathered at this time. The esthetician may be regarded as an additional health-care member who is responsible for the growth of the esthetic practice, and administrative responsibilities may be involved. Larger medical offices may already have an administrator in place. However, the esthetician must realize that extra time and energy must be spent on follow-up of patients who are new to the esthetic portion of the practice, and it may be to the esthetician's advantage to help in the coordination of scheduling these appointments.

Putting together a resumé can be overwhelming and somewhat intimidating for the esthetician just out of esthetics school, and there are ways that you can target your areas of expertise. Perhaps you worked in the past as a medical assistant or you have taken courses in anatomy and physiology or medical terminology. It is important to begin with a good cover letter outlining what you are interested in and why you have approached this physician. Bear in mind that if the physician has not already thought about adding esthetic services to the practice, physicians certainly have been hearing about it at medical meetings. You will need to follow-up on your resumé and try to schedule a time to see the physician. If you have done all of the above and still have not been able to make an appointment, then it is safe to assume that the physician is not interested in esthetic services and that you should focus your energy elsewhere. Remember, not all physicians believe or are interested in adding esthetic services to their practices.

No career changes should be done without careful planning and consideration of your abilities and what you like to do. Ask yourself the following questions:

- ■ Have you taken the time to make a mental list or even written down what you enjoy and the things you really like to do either at work or during your leisure time?

- ■ Have you formulated a clear description of what you think your role will be in a physician's practice?

- ■ Where would you best fit: in a dermatology office, plastic or reconstructive surgery practice, or in a rehabilitation center dealing with burn survivors or other rehabilitation patients?

■ There are several different kinds of resumés: the targeted resumé and the chronological resumé are two. What type works best for you, considering your experience and educational background?

■ Your resumé won't walk in by itself. Have you considered how to effectively introduce it with a cover letter?

❖ Chapter Four ❖

The Interview

Now that you've prepared your tools—your game plan, your job description, your resumé, and your cover letter—it's time to go public with them and set up your interviews.

In this chapter, you will learn:

- how to make initial contact with the physician's office

- how to handle resistance and get past gatekeepers

- how to arrange the first interview

- effective interview techniques

- things to avoid in an interview

Want to Connect?
Use Your Connections

Now comes the hard part—getting the first interview. Rule number one: if someone else can do it for you, let them. Getting the job you want isn't a game, and there's nothing that says you have to do it the hard way. If your friend, uncle, parent, or spouse has a good friend who's a dermatologist or plastic surgeon, you'd be foolish not to ask them to arrange an introduction. In fact, your first step should be to systematically review all the people you know to see if someone has a good relationship with a physician you'd like to work with or knows someone who works in the kind of practice you'd like to join. Don't overlook the obvious. If a family member is a physician or works as a health professional, ask for help. And ask your own family physician or internist for leads. He or she probably has a good relationship with a local dermatologist or plastic surgeon to whom he refers patients; there's no reason your physician shouldn't be able to arrange an appointment for you; if not an actual job interview, you may be able to arrange for an informational interview.

If you can't find someone who can help arrange that first interview, think harder. If you still can't think of anyone, go to step two, arranging it yourself. Unless that first arranged interview turned into a business opportunity, you'd probably have to go to step two anyway.

The First Cold Call—Limiting Your Emotional Exposure

Most people are nervous and uncomfortable calling people they don't know, but arranging an interview needn't be a nerve-wrenching experience. Generally, what makes this kind of call so uncomfortable is that the caller has exaggerated its importance; by the time you've finished thinking about it, the call carries the entire weight of your career decision, of your acceptance by the world at large, of your financial security, and of your entire future.

Step back. This is just a phone call to a stranger who you may never see or care about again. On the other hand, it could work to your favor. Really, it's a win-win situation: you might come away with an appointment for an interview, and the experience, even if it doesn't end with an appointment, will help you develop your technique for the next call. Remember that, important as making calls to set up interviews is, no one call will determine your success or failure. Regardless of the outcome, you'll still have dinner tonight, go to sleep, wake up tomorrow, and life will go on.

Minimizing Your Discomfort

It's perfectly normal to feel a bit uncomfortable making this kind of call, but you can minimize your discomfort if you keep a few things in mind. First, you're not asking anyone for a favor. On the contrary. You have an attractive proposal that you'd like to discuss with the physician you're trying to arrange an appointment with. Until you actually meet, neither of you knows if it will work out to your mutual benefit. The point is, if you can come to a mutually satisfactory arrangement, it will benefit both

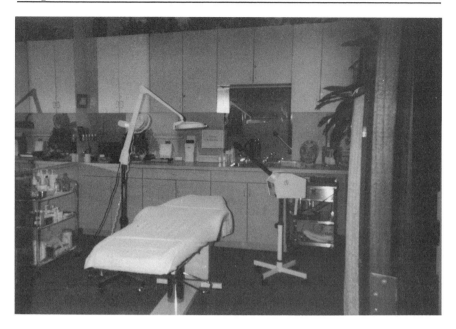

Treatment room in a physician's office

of you. In other words, you're calling with potentially good news, and we rarely get cold feet when we have good news to convey.

Second, remember that you're calling not to get a job but to set up an interview to discuss a profitable business proposal. You don't really know yet if you want to work with this physician. Much as you'll have to sell yourself to the physician, the physician will have to sell you on why his or her practice is a good place to work. At the least, you should expect a courteous response when you call, since anything less could indicate an office in disarray and/or unhappy employees. If that's the case, you're ahead of the game if you don't waste time with that practice. I don't mean to suggest that you should really judge a practice on the basis of the way a single call is answered; there may be a reasonable explanation for a less than pleasant receptionist. But as someone considering establishing a professional relationship with a physician's practice, you are not a supplicant begging for a favor but a skilled professional who is interested in whether or not joining this practice is a reasonable career move.

Third, keep in mind that this is a business call, not a personal call. If the physician has no interest in adding esthetic services to the practice, it's not a personal rejection. We'll talk more about overcoming resistance, but we won't be talking about personal rejection, because it's irrelevant. Some physicians don't want to expand their practices, and some may see no role for an esthetician in their practices, but few physicians, especially in dermatology or plastic surgery, don't respect the role esthetics plays in patients' wellbeing. So not only are they not rejecting you personally, they're not even rejecting your profession. They simply don't want to incorporate your services in their practice.

Know What You Want

Before you actually make your call, make sure you have your objectives clearly in focus. Generally, what you really want is to arrange a meeting with the physician; that should be your primary focus. But it is important to have one or two backup objectives in mind so that if you don't come away with an appointment, you won't come away completely empty-handed. Your secondary objective should be to arrange a time to talk further on the phone. In fact this is the more realistic objective on a first call made during regular office hours, because the chance of being connected directly to the physician probably isn't good, if only because he or she is probably seeing a patient. Finally, be prepared to hear that if you're not calling about a medical problem, no one has time to talk to you. Don't be flustered. Simply ask when would be a better time to call.

Getting Past Gatekeepers

Much has been written for job hunters about getting past corporate secretaries, the people who decide who does and who does not get through to decision makers. Much of this information pertains to large corporations, not professional practices, but some generalities are relevant to your quest, and some information and techniques are unique to physicians' offices.

Before you begin, remember that the primary purpose of the practice is to take care of patients and that people with medical needs come first. That sounds simple, but it can go a long way toward putting into perspective why you may not gain immediate access to the physician. The second thing to remember is that physicians are chronically short of time, which makes the role of gatekeeper important. Receptionists and nurses help physicians maintain their schedules, in so far as that's possible, and help them keep things on track despite the inevitable emergencies. They also prevent patients who tend to use office visits as social occasions from stealing limited time from other patients with genuine medical concerns.

The more efficient you appear, the more attractive you'll be to the physician and the physician's staff. So come to the point immediately when you call. Say who you are and that you'd like to arrange a time to talk to the physician in person about the prospects for adding esthetic services to the practice. If you've already sent your resumé with its cover letter, mention that you're following up to schedule a meeting.

Don't be surprised if the receptionist isn't familiar with the term *esthetician*; simply explain in simple terms what it means— this is not the time for a lengthy description of the fine points of the profession. Physician's offices receive many calls from people who want to see the physician about non-medical issues, usually people who want to sell them something (from medical equipment and office furniture to personal financial services) or persuade them to prescribe a particular drug. By stating right away that you're interested in exploring the possibility of joining the practice, you immediately differentiate yourself from the long list of callers who are strictly interested in making a sale.

It's a good idea to ask if this is a good time to arrange an appointment. Since the receptionist may have to check with the physician and may have to search through an appointment book, this may not be a good time. If it isn't, the receptionist should tell you, and you can ask when would be a convenient time for you to call back. Try to phrase the question positively, "Is this a good time to call to arrange an appointment?" rather than "Is this a bad time?" or "Have I caught you at a bad time?" Phrasing it negatively is an invitation to dismiss you, especially if by *bad* you mean busy or inconvenient; physicians' offices are always busy.

At this point, one of four things can happen. The receptionist may schedule the appointment for you; she may ask you to call back; she may ask you to leave your number and offer to return your call at another time; or she may refuse to help you, perhaps saying the physician isn't interested in adding esthetic services. We don't have to talk about the first option except to mention you should make sure you have the details right by repeating the scheduled time and place and, of course, thanking the receptionist.

If this isn't a good time, offer to call back at a better time. The advantage of calling back, rather than the other way around, is that you are in control; the receptionist could forget to return your call, your message may get lost among the non-medical calls to be returned, or the receptionist may simply not want to deal with you, now or ever. If you ask for a good time to call back, it keeps you in control. A variation on this scenario is that the receptionist says he or she doesn't know whether the physician would be interested in seeing you and that you should call back after office hours and talk directly to the physician. Again, make sure you are clear about when you should call again, and thank the receptionist.

Much more difficult to deal with is the receptionist who doesn't want to make an appointment and doesn't offer to put you through to the physician to let him or her decide whether to see you. How do you turn this reluctant receptionist into an ally? Books on corporate job hunting frequently suggest that you simply elude the gatekeeper and get directly to the decision maker; they often suggest that you manipulate the truth, such as using the boss's first name, implying you're a colleague or a friend, or mounting a sneak attack, such as calling before or after normal business hours when the boss is likely to be in the office but not the gatekeeper. Don't try either tactic. If you do ultimately join the practice, the receptionist will be your colleague, and if your introduction has been based on a falsehood, you may never be able to repair the relationship. The avoidance tactic probably won't work, and even if it did, it's rarely wise to approach a potential employer by surprise; the physician might have answered the phone directly because he or she was expecting a personal call or a call from a patient or colleague. Finding a stranger on the line is unlikely to be a pleasant surprise.

One technique that works surprisingly well when you encounter hostility from a receptionist is to frankly ask for help. Ask if you can call back to talk to her when she has a few minutes, even if she thinks the physician has no interest in your services. Tell her you'd appreciate help in understanding the kind of practice the physician has so you can better target other physi-

cians. Say you'd like to talk about the kinds of patients the practice handles so you can gauge the kind of esthetic services that
type of practice might need. At all times be polite and friendly; if
the receptionist seems short-tempered, it may be because of
something happening in the office, or she just could be in a bad
mood. People generally respond well to a sincere request for
help. Asking for her opinion is flattering, and most people react
well to flattery.

Finally, if nothing else, you can ask if she knows of any
other practices in the area that might be interested in what you
can do. If the receptionist isn't helpful, don't give up. Try calling
again at a different time on a different day; you might get someone else who is more amenable to helping you get an appointment. But if you find you're not getting anywhere, you're probably better off devoting your time and efforts to another practice.

While most physicians' receptionists are trained to screen
calls and assign proper priorities to them, they're rarely told to
prevent someone from getting through at all. You are likely to
either get a time to come in and talk to the physician after office
hours or a time to talk on the phone.

The Phone Mini-Interview

Your first object, of course, is to arrange a meeting. If, however,
you're told to speak with the physician on the phone, you'll
have to use that phone conversation to press for a real interview.

If you haven't already done so, forward your resumé and a
cover letter immediately. The last paragraph of the cover letter
should mention that you look forward to speaking with the
physician at the time and day you've arranged. But because
you've sent your resumé, don't assume the physician has read it.
Your phone interview should serve to very briefly and selectively
reinforce the resumé's main points. The fact that the physician is
taking the time to speak with you suggests a least some degree of
interest, and your purpose is not to fully convince the physician
that you should be a part of his practice—at this point, you don't
know if you really want to join it; rather, you want to arrange a
face-to-face interview.

The Interview—What Physicians Expect, What You Want to Know

All of the preparation—the resumé, the cover letters, the calls—is designed for one thing: to secure an interview with a physician who might be interested in adding your services to his or her practice. Everything so far has been leading up to the interview.

Appearance

As for all interviews, appearance counts; first impressions are lasting impressions, and if they're not positive, they're last impressions. As an esthetician, you're probably more aware of this fact than most people, but that doesn't mean you can take it for granted. The apparel and makeup that mark you as fashionable and stylish in a salon may be entirely inappropriate in a physician's office. That's certainly not to say that you should disregard fashion or ignore flattering makeup at a dermatologist's or plastic surgeon's office, but it does mean that you should be aware that the tone and demeanor likely to make patients comfortable in a medical setting is different from what works in a salon or a nightclub.

Rather than prescribe what specific clothes or makeup you should use, I will provide a few general guidelines. Broadly speaking, the goal should be to achieve an attractive look without calling undue attention to yourself. You should avoid heavy makeup of any kind, overly long fingernails, and extreme hair styles. Moderation is the key. If your outfit would be out of place in a business office, it would be out of place in a physician's office. That's not to say you have to wear dull gray suits; you can be less formal than that, but what you wear should be fairly simple. To put it simply, look like a medical professional, not a model. (I've addressed these remarks to women because men generally have much less to think about when it comes to dressing for work or for an interview; a conservative business suit is the obvious choice.)

The Actual Interview

Your appearance will be completely irrelevant if you fail to appear on time. Arrive early, and if you have to wait, ask the receptionist for any literature the physician distributes to new patients. You can profitably use the time to review these brochures or to go over your resumé and job description (make sure you bring at least two copies of your resumé with you, even if you've sent it ahead) so that you're clear about the key points you want to make.

There are several things to keep in mind about the interview itself. You'll have to ignore some of the standard business interviewing techniques because this isn't a standard business interview. Rather than replying to an advertisement, you initiated the interview; you're proposing that the physician add new services to the practice and that you're the right person to perform them. It's important to remember that it's not at all unlikely that the physician doesn't really know much about esthetic services in general and, even if he or she has had time to review your resumé, very little about what you can really do. Your goal in this interview should be to educate the physician about the field while presenting yourself as a valuable addition to the practice.

If the physician is a man, he may be completely unfamiliar with salon services. If she is a woman, her awareness of what you do is probably limited to her own experience with salon services. In either case, you'll have to talk about the role esthetic services can play in his or her medical practice. This is the time to be assertive. After the usual pleasantries, begin by explaining the concept of medically oriented esthetics. You'll have to differentiate between the usual assumptions about salon services and the specific role certain services can play in the physician's particular practice. Make sure you focus on the medical aspects of the services. In the case of dermatology, you would emphasize your knowledge of noncomedogenic cosmetics, for instance, and your experience with glycolic-acid peels; for plastic surgery, you might talk about your experience using makeup to camouflage various deformities and medical conditions and the role deep cleansing and toning can play in preparation for surgical procedures.

Does that mean you shouldn't talk about the purely esthetic aspect of your work? Of course not. Your skill at making people look their best is extremely valuable to any dermatology or plastic surgery practice. The difference here is that while the primary focus in a salon is making people look good, the primary focus in a medical practice, with the exception of purely cosmetic procedures, is making them well. To the extent that their appearance affects patients' mental health, your work is really part of that primary medical function, although it is only one part of the larger medical picture. You'll also contribute directly to medical care by helping prepare the skin for surgical procedures, helping educate the patient on skin care and the proper use of cosmetics, and perhaps by performing extraction procedures and doing chemical peels.

But the purely cosmetic aspect of what you do is no less valuable, since it adds tremendous value to the purely medical work the physician does. For the plastic surgery patient, learning to properly apply makeup can turn a procedure that makes a difference into one that works a transformation. In fact, your work with these patients will complement the broader job of the surgeon, which is to remold the person's self-image as much as it is to change the structure of tissue and bone. And the things you teach patients will give them a sense of self-determination and mastery that the purely medical procedures can't provide. Don't underestimate the value of this work, but don't assume the physician is aware of its importance; some physicians are very sensitive to their patients' concerns about their appearance; others are not, and some are simply uncomfortable when they venture beyond the purely medical into the psychological.

You can be invaluable to the physician's practice in taking on some of the responsibility for patients' emotional wellbeing, both by focusing on the cosmetic implications of surgical and medical procedures and by being another person to whom patients can confide their concerns, hopes, and fears. Try during the interview to talk about how you've helped salon clients feel better about themselves, and if you can think of any cases in which this has led to significant changes in their lives, by all means describe your role in helping bring them about. This after all is one of the ways you find your work satisfying, and you should make the physician aware that your interest in people goes beyond simply showing them how to look good.

Avoid exaggerated claims. Physicians undergo scientific as well as clinical training, and they will respond poorly to you if they think you're unduly influenced by the latest fad. While advertisers tout the benefits of "natural" products, physicians know that bacteria are natural and that the body can't tell the difference between a molecule of vitamin C that comes from a lab and one that comes from an orange. And they are aware that no cosmetic procedure can cure or even mask a deep psychological disorder, so don't suggest that you can turn a recluse into a social butterfly with a simple makeover. Rather, try to convey an understanding of how esthetics relates to larger issues of medicine and psychological wellbeing. Acne, for instance, plays an important role in any dermatology practice. You should be able to demonstrate an awareness of common cosmetic ingredient allergies, contact dermatitis, sun damage, and seborrhea. Other skin diseases are other common complaints, so you should be able to talk about them. Plastic surgeons will be particularly concerned about the process of skin aging, wound healing, scarring, and the uses of camouflage makeup. Obviously, if these topics are unfamiliar to you, you should spend time learning about them before your interview by consulting standard texts on medical esthetics, college-level texts on health, and professional esthetic journals.

An effective way to demonstrate your skills and the kind of work you do is to offer to give the physician a demonstration session at your salon or in the office if you're not working at a salon. If the physician has never had a facial treatment, your demonstration can be a real eye-opener. In any case, it will serve to convince the physician of your skill and understanding of effective techniques. It also puts you in the role of an authority figure in a way that's nonthreatening to the physician. Some physicians, especially men, may be uncomfortable serving as the subject. In that case, offer to treat the receptionist or nurse and invite the physician to watch the procedure. Actually working on the physician or one of his assistants gives you the chance to prove what you say you can do, and it can go a long way toward convincing the physician that you really can add value to a medical practice.

The Follow-Up Letter

One more part of the interview is important: the follow-up letter. It's tempting to let it go, to rely on the good impression you've made and the intention to call back in a few days. But it would be a mistake to miss the opportunity to reinforce the positive points you've made during the interview. A follow-up letter does not need to be elaborate; even a simple thank-you note is much better than no letter at all. At the least, your letter should thank the physician for taking the time to see you, and it should reiterate your interest in joining the practice, if you have decided you would, in fact, like to, or further exploring how you can work together if you're still not sure it's the right spot for you. If the two of you found areas of common interest, mention that, if only to say something like "I found your emphasis on the importance of learning the right way to clean the skin very interesting, since it has always been a key part of my continuing education programs at the salon."

❧ Review and Summary ❧

When you have made it as far as the interview you have established the physician's interest in meeting with you and discussing options for adding esthetic services to his or her practice. If you have already established the interest through your resumé and cover letter you should feel comfortable going in and presenting yourself as a professional who could enhance the care of patients in this medical practice. Cold calling can certainly be very difficult and is not always the best approach for trying to "sell" your services to the physician. It can be difficult to get past the gatekeeper or the receptionist of the practice, and certainly making that person an ally is to your advantage.

An important point to remember is that the term *esthetician* is not well known to physicians and therefore explanation of the term may be necessary to obtain the interview. With so many people using terms *clinical esthetician, paramedical esthetician,* and *clinical specialist,* it may be confusing to the physician when you call. In order to effectively talk about your credentials, it is always advisable to bring along extra copies of your resumé and license so that you can leave a copy with the physician.

The day of the interview, first impressions are the best impressions. Arrive looking like a professional. This image will help to secure the physician's interest. Arrive on time, even though you may have to wait a few minutes if the physician is in the middle of patient hours. Arriving ten or fifteen minutes early will give you the time to observe the practice and take a moment to look at the literature available in the waiting room. By reviewing the literature available to patients you will obtain a fair idea of the types of services the physician now offers. From this information you can determine the types of treatments and services that the physician may be interested in adding. Then your common sense comes into play, listening to the physician about needs in the particular practice. Learning what the physician is presently doing in the office can also better prepare you for what areas you will need to discuss.

During the interview you should take notes, particularly if the physician is interested in procedures that you do and has requested additional information. A follow-up letter will indicate your level of professionalism in providing the information that the physician requested, or the letter may be a simple note thanking the physician for the time even if he or she was not interested in incorporating esthetic treatments.

Cold calls to secure a job interview can be uncomfortable— are they always necessary? Ask yourself the following questions:

- Have you thought of who you know who has connections with the practices in which you might want to work?

- When you can't avoid cold calling, have you done everything to put the call into perspective, to limit your emotional exposure?

- Have you clearly stated to yourself the real objective to your call?

- Have you formulated a plan to deal with the receptionist?

- Have you rehearsed your thoughts, indicating the benefits of adding esthetic services to the physician's practice?

- Have you considered offering the physician a complimentary treatment?

Chapter Five

The Employment Agreement

Over the years I have had the opportunity to sit in on numerous salary negotiations, and I have seen the same mistake made over and over again. The offer of employment is put on the table, all the details are outlined, and the prospective employee, without a moment's hesitation, responds. Whether the response was positive or negative, it was not thought out. An employment agreement is a commitment that you, as the employee, will have to live with for the term of the agreement.

In this chapter you will learn:

- to examine the issues before you accept the job offer

- salary and benefits considerations

- the job description

- the duration of the agreement

- the advantages and disadvantages of working as an employee or an independent contractor

- accepting or rejecting the offer

- how to determine your worth to the medical practice

Congratulations! Your interview concluded with a job offer. You've enjoyed a moment of triumph, a top-of-the-world rush.

Now what?

I don't want to spoil the fun, but you've got some critical decisions to make, and this is no time to sit back and rest on your laurels. Negotiating your employment agreement is perhaps the most important part of the job search, because how well you do it will largely determine how happy you'll be in the job you've taken great pains to secure. In fact, in my experience, perhaps the single most destructive thing estheticians do when they move into a new job, especially when they change career directions by entering a medical practice, is they neglect the negotiating process altogether. That's not unique to estheticians. An amazing number of job applicants in all fields, delighted by the triumph of getting a firm job offer, simply accept the job without even knowing what they're agreeing to beyond their base salary. That's a sure strategy for disappointment at best and, in some cases, real trouble with lasting regrets.

Fortunately, that won't happen to you because you'll go into your interview well prepared to negotiate the terms of your employment.

Do I Really Have to Negotiate?

Many people find the whole idea of negotiating with a prospective employer intimidating, and the first instinct is to avoid anything unpleasant. There are two situations in which you can entirely skip the negotiating process: when the offer is wildly better than anything you could have anticipated or when the offer is clearly a fair one and you're not greedy. If the physician follows the job offer with something like "I was thinking of starting you at 50 dollars an hour; how does that sound?" You probably don't have much to think about. Although if that's the first offer, maybe you should push for 75 dollars! Let's get back to reality again. If the offer is 15 dollars an hour plus benefits, it's probably fair, and you would be entirely reasonable to simply accept it. There's no rule that says you have to negotiate.

Often, the initial offer is on the low end of a reasonable scale. Here's where you probably should negotiate, even if negotiation isn't your favorite activity. Most employers go into the process knowing the upper figure they're willing to pay, but they don't make this their first offer; they start with a figure closer to the least they think the prospective employee will accept. If you simply agree, you'll be shortchanging yourself. Don't be intimidated by the fear that if you don't accept the first figure the whole offer will be withdrawn. If you're being offered the job, there's always room to talk about salary and benefits. The only way you'll wind up losing the job altogether is if you take an inflexible, unyielding approach to negotiating and then proceed to make unreasonable demands. But that's one of the best ways to make yourself unwanted in just about any situation.

Assuming you will negotiate the terms of your employment, the best way to proceed is to deal with one issue at a time, always keeping in mind that the real economic value of the job will be a sum of all the parts, including salary, benefits, and the time you'll spend working.

Salary

When it comes to negotiating the terms of a job offer, most people concentrate on salary. Other parts of your compensation, such as health and liability insurance, profit sharing, or retirement plans, are important, but your salary is probably the key to determining whether or not the job offer is worthwhile. Just bear in mind that, important as it is, salary isn't everything. To evaluate what a job is worth in financial terms, you have to look at the entire package.

The first rule of salary negotiation is to recognize that whatever salary you wind up accepting will pretty much be your salary for the foreseeable future. It is a grave mistake to accept a salary that you consider too low in the hope that once your employer sees what a great asset you are, your salary will go up. It might, but not by much. Annual raises, remember, tend to be a percentage increase of your current salary, and if that figure is low, the real amount of any raise will be proportionately low. Start out too low, and the only way you will make what you should is to start the process all over again with another job.

Now is the time to negotiate the best salary possible. Remember that negotiating the salary you want is a continuation of the process of selling yourself to the physician as a valued addition to the practice. That's what you've been doing all along in pursuing this job, and so far you've been successful. There's no reason why you shouldn't be successful in the negotiation process as well. But it's unlikely you'll get what you want unless you know what that is. Everyone would like to earn a six-figure salary, of course, and seven figures would be even better. But before going any further, let's talk reality.

The points of your salary negotiation will be determined by the usual factors of supply and demand and by how much you're likely to contribute to the physician's bottom line. Fortunately, the supply side of the equation, how many other people have applied for your job, is less important in this profession than in most other work situations, since this is a relatively new field and there probably aren't many people applying for the position you're considering. On the other hand, because this is a new field and physicians aren't knowledgeable about how much estheticians in medical practices earn, there are no well-established salary guidelines. When salary standards don't exist, negotiations can be more difficult. And since physicians generally don't have a clear idea of what the incremental revenue potential is for adding esthetic services, it can be difficult for them to know what a reasonable salary might be.

This means you'll have to come prepared not only with a clear idea of what you want to earn but with some estimate of what additional revenue the practice can reasonably expect to make if it hires you. There is no exact formula for determining how much revenue an esthetician will bring to a medical practice, because it will vary with the type of practice and locations since prices for both esthetic services and medical procedures vary quite widely throughout the country. As a rough guide, I've calculated some of the basic costs of providing esthetic services.

Treatment Cost

Treatment costs can be divided into three categories: laundry, miscellaneous sundries, and actual product to be used. Laundry items for pickup and delivery each week would consist of fresh linens, hand towels, patient gowns, and thermal blankets. The costs for these items vary state to state, but below is the average.

Laundry

1 Fitted Sheet	$0.55
1 Flat Sheet	.55
2 Terry Towels	.50
1 Gown	.90
1 Blanket	2.95
Subtotal	**$5.45**

Sundries

Sundry items are the costs of cotton swabs, combine strips, applicators, etc. To determine these costs you need to refer to your inventory book, which should be up-to-date with the most recent prices, and determine what you would need to administer the treatments.

---

1 Scoppette	$0.15
2 cotton pads 2x2	.02
2 gauze pads 4x4	.06
2 combine strips	.15
1 pair gloves	.16
1 medicine cup	.02
1 distilled water	.13
1 lancet	.09
6 tissues	.02
Subtotal	**$0.80**

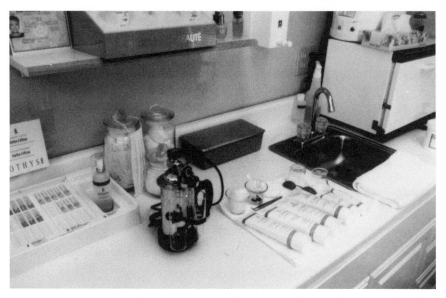

Part of the total cost of a treatment is the cost of the products used in that treatment.

Product

Again, refer to your inventory book and come up with the cost for the amount you would use for this type of treatment.

Cleanser	$0.62
Glycolic Acid	2.50
Mask	1.93
Sunscreen	.10
Subtotal	**$5.15**

Laundry costs	$5.45
Sundry costs	.80
Product costs	$5.15
Total costs	$11.40
Average hourly wage of esthetician	$14.00
Total average cost (excluding rent overhead and office staff)	**$25.40**

Add the three columns together $5.45 + .80 + $5.15, to bring the total to $11.40. Add in your hourly wage; in this case it was averaged to $14.00 an hour. The grand total equals $25.40. Keep in mind that this excludes the rental overhead of the treatment room that you are using and other overhead costs, such as the reception-ist who books appointments and support staff. Therefore in order to make a profit of a least 50 percent on this service, you would need to charge a minimum of $50.00 for the service.

The general rule of thumb I've found that works is to use the physician's fee schedule as a guide. For instance, if the physi-cian charges $60 for a fifteen-minute follow-up visit, it would work well to charge the same amount for a one-hour visit with the esthetician. Additional services such as eye treatments, hand treatments, lymphatic drainage treatments, chemical exfoliations, etc., could then be added-on service fees. The bottom line is that you want to have the treatment room profitable every hour.

Product Sales

The most overlooked revenue producer by physicians is product sales. As long as I've been an esthetician I've realized that I can physically only see thirty-five to forty patients per week. I wasn't going to get anywhere by simply doing service after service. The real money lies in the sale of products. This idea may instill fear and apprehension in the physician, and this will be discussed more in Chapter Eight, but the reality is, with-out product sales, the profitability of this venture will fail. Let's take a look at the facts.

Let's say you sell one product at a retail cost of $20.00 to twenty patients per month. That's a total gross income of $400.00 X 12 months, or $4,800. The additional income to the practice would be $2400 assuming you do a 100 percent markup on the product. (For instance, the wholesale cost of the product was $10.00, and it was retailed at $20.00, or a 50 percent profit on the retail price.)

Product Sales
Average Product Sale of $20.00
(that's selling one product to 20 patients per month)

$20 X 20 Patients	$400.00
Gross product sales	$4800.00
Net profit to practice	**$2400.00**

Salary versus Total Compensation

The other side of this issue is knowing what you really want and need in terms of salary. Those are actually two different things. There's probably a minimum amount you need to support yourself (I assume that you're working because you need to, whether or not there's another income in your household) and a minimum amount you need to earn in order to feel that you're not being taken advantage of. You should concentrate on the latter figure in most cases; it's always a serious mistake to accept a salary that makes you resent going to work each day. Knowing the figure you absolutely must get to accept the job is important because it gives you an idea of where to lead the discussions ahead of time, no matter how nervous you might be and how attractive the job may seem.

During the actual salary negotiations, your attitude can be crucial in determining both the outcome and the way your future employer sees you. Don't see the process as a competition; see it as an opportunity to explore your prospective position and its benefits both to you and to the physician. Keep in mind all of the ways in which you can add value to the practice by performing procedures not done now by the physician, by adding new services (and revenue), by selling products, and by bringing new patients to the practice through referrals and simply because the practice now offers new services it couldn't provide without you. Be positive. The best answer to objections that a salary request is too high is to point out the extra value you bring to the practice and the extra revenue that will accrue to it as a result. The idea is to let the physician know at all times that you think this can be a win-win situation; an opportunity for you to practice esthetics in a setting that will bring you immense rewards and an opportunity for the physician to offer valued services to his or her patients and to increase the practice's income in the process.

There are three possible outcomes to the salary negotiation process: you get the salary you've asked for; the salary you're offered is simply too low and you decide not to accept the job; the salary is lower than you'd like but not so low that, given the right combination of non-salary items (benefits, bonus, vacation time, shorter work hours), you could be happy with the job. As I mentioned above, knowing your bottom limit is important because there's no sense wasting time—yours or the physician's—

if you're not going to be happy with the compensation. If, on the other hand, the offer that emerges from your discussion of salary is less than you'd like but not out of an acceptable range, the next step is to talk about the other, non-salary, aspects of the job offer. Even if the salary is right, you'll have to talk about issues such as benefits, vacation, bonuses, and retirement plans.

Beyond Salary—Negotiating Benefits and Other Non-Salary Compensation

Your salary will be just one part of your compensation. In fact, your benefits, such as a health insurance and retirement plans, may be almost as important from an economic standpoint as your actual salary. Here, there is sometimes less room for negotiation, at least when it comes to health insurance and retirement plans. The reason for this is that an employer may not offer one insurance plan to some people in the office and a different one to others. It is even illegal for the physician to provide a "Cadillac" plan for himself/herself and a "Chevy" plan for the employees. Everyone must be offered the same basic plan. In some cases, the employee may elect to buy additional coverage, but the basic plan must be the same for all employees of the corporation (most medical practices are organized as professional corporations).

Medical Insurance

When it comes to medical insurance, I've noticed that estheticians moving into a medical practice can make several serious mistakes. They are usually fairly young and healthy, so they discount the need for good medical insurance. In fact, anyone at any time can suddenly become a major consumer of medical services, either through an unforeseen illness or as a result of an accident.

The second mistake is to assume that because you'll be working for a physician, your medical needs will be taken care of. You may get a free flu shot each year, but don't assume you will get free medical care. In the first place, it's almost always a very bad idea to let your employer act as your physician. It confuses the roles of employer and employee and compromises the objectivity essential to proper medical care. Furthermore, even if your employer actually provides certain medical services to you, as a dermatologist or plastic surgeon, his or her area of expertise will be limited. If you need the care of an internist, gynecologist, or any other specialty, you'll be out of luck. And don't count on the physician's network of referring physicians. They may see the physician or the physician's family as a courtesy, but that courtesy rarely if ever extends beyond the range of the physician's immediate family, if it extends that far. Furthermore, with the proliferation of health maintenance organizations (HMOs) and other managed care systems that are taking over medical care, even these courtesies are becoming a thing of the past.

In other words, you'll need to look at the health insurance plan the practice offers with the same care as you would look at a plan offered by a salon or any other business. The key questions are: Is it an HMO or PPO plan, or does it offer you unrestricted choice of physicians and hospitals? What are the deductibles? What are the benefit limits? What services are covered, and what are not? Will the practice pay the entire premium, or will you have to pick up some of it yourself? Does the plan offer dental coverage? If so, how much? If you haven't dealt with these questions in a previous job or as an independent purchaser of health insurance, you'll need to educate yourself about these issues before you even get to the interview stage. They're important, and they will be an important element in deciding whether the job offer is good or bad. A good salary with no health-insurance benefits or with inadequate benefits may be a bad deal.

On the other hand, you may already have an insurance plan that you've been paying for on your own and are satisfied. If you want to continue with the plan you already have, and if the practice offers its employees another plan, you might very well suggest that, since you won't be participating in the practice's plan, you'd like to receive whatever the plan pays for its employees' insurance premiums as additional compensation. Since the practice planned to spend that much on your premiums, asking for it as additional salary is entirely reasonable. You should be aware, however, that the additional income will be taxed along with the rest of your salary. While the amount is relatively small compared to the rest of your salary, depending on your total income from this job and from outside sources, it might be enough to push you into a different tax bracket.

The other benefit estheticians pay too little attention to is retirement plans. You'll notice, I haven't used the term "fringe benefit" when talking about insurance and retirement plans; that's because it's a terrible mistake to think of these plans as anything but integral parts of your total compensation. What looks like an "extra" to a healthy person of twenty-six looks very different to the man or woman of fifty-six. But when you're fifty-six or if you are unfortunate enough to develop a serious illness or be involved in an accident, it will be too late to start thinking of these issues. A financial adviser once gave me this advice: at the age of thirty you should have saved approximately $30,000 for retirement. That means that money should be in a tax-deferred retirement plan such as an IRA, unavailable except in the most serious emergencies until you reach at least the age of fifty-nine. Each year, you should add another $2,000. All too often, I hear the line, "My husband takes care of that." Grow up. Business and professional men and women need to take care of themselves, regardless of their marital or romantic attachments.

Retirement Plans

There are many types of retirement plans, and I'm not qualified to advise you on the pros and cons of each. Some plans are called "defined benefit plans". As their name implies, these plans offer specific benefits, such as a guaranteed income when the employee retires, usually at age sixty-five. They're more typical of large corporations, and even in these, they are often no longer offered. Some plans are defined contribution plans; profit-sharing plans fall into this category because the employer (the practice, in this case) contributes a set percent of profits to accounts owned by employees. These plans may or may not be retirement plans. If you're not familiar with the general kinds of retirement and profit-sharing plans that you're likely to encounter, take some time to educate yourself about them. An hour or two spent with any of the popular books on managing your finances will be well worth the effort.

You need to know these things regardless of the kind of job you take, but knowing about them before you negotiate your compensation package is particularly important. As I mentioned, a very attractive package of employer-paid health insurance, profit sharing, and retirement plans can often compensate for a salary that's on the low end of what's fair. But you have to be careful not to accept a salary offer assuming that these benefits will make up the difference between completely inadequate and fair. A salary is paid every week or biweekly. Profit sharing depends on the profits of the practice, and it is paid just once a year, and retirement benefits, important as they are for your overall economic health, won't pay the mortgage or the car payments.

Other Issues

Other issues you'll want to discuss are vacation, tuition reimbursement, overtime policies, sick leave, and disability and liability insurance. The important thing is not to assume anything; discuss these things openly so there won't be any misunderstanding later. And, again, don't assume these things aren't important just because they haven't been in the past. Tuition reimbursement, or subscriptions to journals for instance, may not have been an issue while you worked in a salon, but you may find that you want to upgrade your medical knowledge now that you'll be working in a physician's office. And while you've been healthy in the past, you must not overlook the possibility, no matter how remote it seems, that you could get sick. If you do, will you be paid from the day you get sick? When will you become eligible for disability insurance? How much insurance will you have, and when will long-term disability payments begin and for how long?

The office may have a set policy about vacation time, and you should know what it is. Often, vacations have to be coordinated with the physician's schedule, especially in one-person practices. If the physician takes an annual two-week vacation in March, does that mean you have to take your vacation then, too? Will you get your full vacation this year, or do you have to work a certain number of months before you can take time off? Sometimes you can negotiate for additional vacation time as compensation for a salary you consider too low, and sometimes you can offer to take additional vacation without pay, but these things need to be agreed upon before you actually accept the position. Also, don't overlook personal days. These may be used for religious holidays or for important personal business. Does the practice offer such days, and if so how many?

Liability insurance is an often overlooked factor during employment negotiations. Don't assume that in the case of a lawsuit you'll be covered by the physician's malpractice insurance. More on this subject in Chapter Six.

Employee or Private Contractor?

In discussing compensation I should deal briefly with the issues of working as an employee versus a private contractor. In most situations, the esthetician is the employee of a physician or medical practice, and this book is geared mainly to those situations in which the esthetician works under the supervision of a physician, part-time or full-time, in a medical practice. In some cases, however, estheticians want to establish their own esthetic practices and team up with a physician, usually with a dermatologist, for referrals for strictly non-medical esthetic services. In this situation, it may be advantageous to organize yourself as an independent business.

The IRS has complex rules, with approximately twenty criteria, to determine whether an individual is an employee or an independent contractor. You can boil them down to several key requirements for determining independent status.

IRS Twenty Factors for Determining Independent or Employee Status

1. **Instruction:** Is the worker told what must be done and how to accomplish the task?

2. **Training:** An employee often receives training. An independent contractor uses his/her own methods.

3. **Integration:** Is the success of the business dependent, to a large degree, upon the worker's performance?

4. **Services Rendered Personally:** An employee renders services personally.

5. **Hiring Assistants:** An employee works for an employer who hires, supervises, and pays workers. An independent contractor would do these functions himself or herself.

6. **Continuing Relationship:** An employer generally has a continuing relationship with an employee.

7. **Set Hours of Work:** An employee generally has hours set by his or her employer. An independent contractor sets his or her own hours.

8. **Full Time Required:** An independent contractor is free to work when and for whom he or she chooses.

9. **Doing Work on Employer Premises:** Off-premise working indicates some independence.

10. **Order of Sequence Set:** An employee generally is given direction as to the order of work to be performed.

11. **Oral or Written Reports:** Reports indicate employer-employee relationship.

12. **Payments:** Payments by the job or on a straight commission basis generally indicates independent contractor status.

13. **Expenses:** An employee's business and travel expenses are generally paid by the employer.

14. **Tools and Materials:** An employer usually furnishes tools and supplies to an employee, but not to an independent contractor.

15. **Investment:** The more investment, the more likely independent contractor status exists.

16. **Profit or Loss:** An independent contractor can make a profit or suffer a loss.

17. **Working for More Than One Firm:** One firm indicates employee status; multiple firms indicate independent contractor status.

18. **Offers Services to General Public:** An independent contractor offers services to the general public.

19. **Right to Fire:** An employee can be fired by an employer.

20. **Right to Quit:** An employee can quit the job at any time without incurring liability.

Reprinted with permission Wilson, L.: Employee or Independant Contractor *PCI Journal of Progressive Clinical Insights* (1995),3:5;16–17.

There are other concerns. If the office has a receptionist, and virtually all medical offices do, it's essential that the receptionist's services to the esthetician be billed separately. If the esthetician is using the medical office phone number for business purposes such as to book appointments, phone charges must be billed separately, not as part of the rent. The esthetician will also have to maintain general and professional liability insurance (the need for insurance as an employee will be discussed in Chapter Six). And this is by no means an exhaustive list. If you plan to set up as an independent contractor you really need the advice of an accountant or health attorney. Several new bills have been proposed and passed in Congress that contain guidelines or "safe harbors" of the types of business arrangements that physicians can make. Ignorance of the law is no defense! Don't try to do it yourself unless you think IRS audits are a fun way to spend your vacation.

As for the economic issues of working as an independent contractor compared to those as an employee, they can be deceptively attractive, but before you make a decision, look at the real, final numbers.

Independent Contractor Weekly Financials

Gross income	$500.00
Taxes (30 percent of gross income)	– $150.00
Health insurance premium	– $62.50
IRA or SEP plan (8 percent of gross income)	– $40.00
Total take home pay (per week)	**$247.50**

Let's assume that your gross income as a private contractor is $500 per week. Now deduct 30 percent for taxes, or $150. Sound high? Perhaps you forgot that as an independent contractor, you're responsible for your entire Social Security tax, not just half as when you work as an employee. Now deduct $62.50 for your health-insurance premium, a reasonable amount based on a plain-vanilla package, which costs $250 a month. Next, deduct $40 for an IRA or SEP plan, a contribution to your retirement of just 8 percent of your income. Once you've finished with all the deductions, you are left with take-home pay of $247.50 per week, or an hourly rate of just $6.18. Paid vacation? Forget it. Sick leave? Again, no way.

I'm not saying there are never situations when you might be better off as an independent contractor, but for the most part, estheticians working in a medical setting are better off as employees.

Duties and Responsibilities— The Job Description

Of course, there's more to a job than getting paid. If you have read Chapter One and done the exercises I recommended there, you know that this is the kind of work you want to do, so you should assume you'll enjoy doing it. But you need to discuss with the physician exactly what you'll be doing and how your day will be organized. The two of you should agree on a specific **job description**. No job description can spell out exactly what you'll be doing every minute of every working day, but a good description should detail the major duties and responsibilities in some detail.

In addition to the duties and responsibilities, the job description may spell out the requirements for the position. This may include a current esthetician's license in states where licensing exists; a certificate or letter of liability insurance coverage (more about this in Chapter Six); a current training and certification in first aid and CPR, although these are usually optional.

It is a good idea to review a copy of the job description, sign it, and keep a copy for yourself. If the physician hasn't actually written such a description, you might suggest that you'd be happier knowing in writing what was expected of you. It really is good business practice to have something in writing that spells out what's expected of you. If nothing's written yet, at least agree verbally on the main points and get one written and okayed by the physician within a reasonable period of your starting date. Save copies of everything you discuss with the physician, and, remember, it's always a good idea to keep written notes of meetings and to memo the physician if any major decisions were agreed upon that affect you or your work habits. The general rule is to get it in writing so you have a record of it!

Sample Job Description

Position: Esthetician

Summary: Responsible for performing skin-care services for patients under the supervision of a physician. Assisting in patient care through communication with office staff and the physician.

Responsibilities:

1. Coordinates patient care with the physician, including but not limited to the use of oral and topical medications, pre- and postoperative care, and various patient compliance concerns.

2. Provides new patients with complimentary consultations regarding skin-care services.

3. Serves as a liaison with the patient coordinator during the pre- and post-operative phase of patient treatment to ensure understanding of the outcome.

4. Maintains treatment rooms and work stations in compliance with OSHA standards.

5. Seeks advice of physician on treatment protocols and advises physician of patient noncompliance.

6. Maintains and insures current patient records detailing treatment procedures, products, medications, and educational information.

7. Takes care of equipment for proper operation, including cleaning, as suggested by manufacturer.

8. Overviews and updates office personnel telephone procedure on handling scheduling, confirming appointments, wait listing, cancellation protocols, and patient tracking.

9. Participates and attends in-service programs and staff meetings.

10. Assists with orientation and training of new office personnel, including but not limited to product education, sales procedures, skin-care services, and any other related protocols.

11. Coordinates any correspondence/brochures to patients regarding their skin-care treatments, product usage, and home-care instructions.

12. Tracks outside referral sources and sends thank-you letters and/or post-consultation letters if referred by another physician.

13. Maintains inventory system for professional and retail products and tracking of sales tax.

14. Orders and stocks medical supplies and products as needed for maintaining treatment room and retail shelves.

Terms of Employment

Even marriages made in heaven don't always last forever. But even if they did, you should know if there's a provisional period during which you can be fired without cause, what, if any, escape clauses exist for the physician (what if the practice proves less profitable than was assumed, what if your services don't produce the incremental revenue the physician was expecting?), and what restrictions will you be subject to after you leave the practice. These non-compete agreement clauses vary in legality from state to state, and you should check with an attorney to see what restrictions are enforceable for you.

You might well be asked to sign a confidentiality or non-disclosure agreement. As an employee of a medical practice, you will be expected to vigorously uphold patients' right to privacy. That's not what I'm talking about here. In an employment agreement, a confidentiality agreement refers to the fact that all information about the practice—names and addresses of patients, for instance, or details about specific treatment procedures or diseases—must remain strictly confidential even after you leave the practice. Patient confidentiality is of utmost importance, especially if you're performing procedures on any famous personalities. It is not appropriate to share with your friends that evening over drinks the details of who, what, and where you treated in the practice that day. Any such disclosures need to be agreed to and signed by the patient.

Sample Employment Contract

Not every practice has a sample **employment contract** made up, although when I assist physicians in setting up esthetic services in their practices, I always suggest that they write one and have the esthetician sign a copy. It protects the physician, and it protects the esthetician from misunderstandings later on. In any case, here's a sample that's typical of the agreements I suggest physicians use. Of course, this is not legally binding in all states, and you need to check with an attorney in your state. The particular practice you plan to join may not use every clause in this sample, but it covers most of the issues you're likely to encounter. It can also serve as a complete guide to the issues you'll want to cover before you actually agree to join a practice.

SAMPLE EMPLOYMENT AGREEMENT

Jane Doe, M.D. (hereinafter referred to as "Doe"), doing business at 123 Main Street, Anton, New York, and Maryanne Smith (hereinafter referred to as "Smith"), residing at 7 Elm Street, Anton, New York, in consideration of the mutual promises made herein, agree to the following:

I. TERM OF EMPLOYMENT

Doe hereby employs Smith, and Smith hereby accepts employment with Doe as an esthetician, commencing on September 26, 1996. The employment shall be for an unspecified period of time and terminable at the will of either party with 30 days notice.

II. DUTIES OF EMPLOYEE

A. Smith shall serve as an esthetician for Doe. In that capacity, Smith shall comply with and perform all acts necessary to discharge her duties including, but not limited to, those relating to esthetic treatments.

(Outline of esthetic treatment/procedures should be attached at this point; refer to Chapter Two.)

B. Smith shall, at her own expense, obtain and maintain in effect malpractice insurance that provides at least $100,000 in liability coverage.

C. The parties contemplate that Smith shall work three days totally, approximately twenty-four hours, at the commencement of her employment, gradually increasing to full-time employment. The pay scale increase will be as follows:

Increase to Four Days—$400.00 or approximately 30 hours,

Increase to Five Days—$500.00 or approximately 40 hours.

However, Doe at all times shall have the sole discretion to increase or decrease the required number of hours or work per week, consistent with the needs of its practice, but Smith must be guaranteed a minimum income of $250.00 per week.

D. The parties acknowledge and agree that, as business needs arise, Smith may have to assume additional responsibilities consistent with this agreement, which have not been expressly set forth herein.

III. DUTIES OF EMPLOYER

Doe shall provide training in the medical aspects of Smith's work. Doe will furnish space, equipment, and supplies necessary for Smith to perform her duties under this Agreement. It is the intent of the parties that Doe and Smith will, in consultation with each other, select the types of services to be offered to Doe's patients, including but not limited to the treatment procedures and the products to be used.

Sample Employment Agreement; check with your legal counsel for one which specifically fits your needs.

IV. COMPENSATION

Doe shall pay Smith as outlined in Section II, Paragraph C, in consideration for the services and covenants contained herein.

B. Performance Bonus

To be based on the sale of over-the-counter and cosmetic products only. This bonus will be 3 percent of Gross Product Receipts for the entire month and will be payable at this time.

C. Vacation Days:

Three days paid vacation (based on present three-day work week)

Four days paid vacation (based on increased four-day work week)

Five days paid vacation (based on increased five-day work week)

**(2) One week (or five days) unpaid vacation may be taken the first year.

(2) One week (or five days) paid vacation may be taken the second year.

D. Benefits:

(i)   Health insurance,

(ii) Profit sharing plan,

(iii) Six paid holidays per year to include; Christmas Day, New Year's Day, Thanksgiving, Independence Day, Labor Day, Memorial Day.

V. CONFIDENTIAL INFORMATION

A. The parties acknowledge and agree that during the term of this contract and in the course of discharging her duties hereunder, Smith will have access to, and become acquainted with, information concerning Doe's operations, including without limitation its current and future business plans, the identities and peculiar needs of its patients, and the manner in which it markets its services. Such information is owned by Doe and regularly used in the operation of its business. This information constitutes Doe confidential, trade secret, proprietary information which confers a competitive advantage to Doe in the operation of its business.

B. Smith agrees that she will not disclose any such confidential information, directly or indirectly, to any other person or entity or use such information (including patients' names and addresses) in any way to the detriment of Doe, either during the term of this contract or at any time thereafter.

VI. UNFAIR COMPETITION

Smith acknowledges and agrees that the sale or unauthorized use of disclosure of any of Doe confidential or proprietary information obtained by Smith during the course of her employment constitutes unfair competition. Smith promises and agrees not to engage in any unfair competition with Doe at any time, whether during or following her employment with Doe.

Sample Employment Agreement; check with your legal counsel for one which specifically fits your needs.

VII. NON-SOLICITATION OF PATIENTS

Smith agrees that she will not solicit the business of any patient of Doe or otherwise attempt to interfere or divert business from Smith either for her own benefit or for the benefit of any other person or business. This duty to refrain from solicitation shall continue for the maximum period allowed by law after the termination of Smith's employment.

VIII. ENTIRE AGREEMENT

This agreement supersedes any and all prior agreements, either oral or written, between the parties with respect to Smith's employment by Doe and contains all of the covenants and agreements between the parties with respect to that employment.

IX. AMENDMENT AND MODIFICATION

This Agreement may only be amended or modified in writing, signed by the parties hereto.

X. SEVERABILITY

If any provision of this Agreement or the application thereof to any party or circumstance shall be determined to be invalid or unenforceable, the remaining provisions of this Agreement shall be not affected and shall be enforced to the fullest extent of the law.

XI. GOVERNING LAW

This Agreement was made and entered into in _____. Each party acknowledges that any breach of this Agreement will cause injury to the other party in _____, and each agrees that the laws of the State of _____ shall apply to any dispute arising hereunder.

Dated:_____By

_____

Jane Doe, M.D.

Dated:_____By

_____

Maryanne Smith

Sample Employment Agreement; check with your legal counsel for one which specifically fits your needs.

The Intangibles

Once you've discussed salary and benefits, are both clear about what will be expected of you, and all the concrete issues have been dealt with, there remain certain intangible concepts that may profoundly influence whether or not you'll be happy as a member of this practice. Don't ignore them simply because they're more difficult to define. If you've come this far, you've probably determined that you're comfortable with the physician and you like what you can see of his or her practice, but you should consider some of the issues that touch on the physician's philosophy of patient care and how the physician will relate to you in a medical setting.

One of the best ways to determine whether you'll really be comfortable working in a practice is to spend a few days there before you make your final commitment. If several physicians are working in the practice, you many want to arrange to work with each of them for a few hours.

Finally, lifestyle and personality issues may affect your relationship with the physician and with the practice. These aren't easy to evaluate precisely, but most of us know what kinds of work habits make us comfortable, and you should try to see if the physician you'll be working with makes you feel comfortable or not. I assume you enjoy working hard, but some physicians are workaholics, and that may not be to your liking. Physicians are usually careful and concerned about details, but this can become obsessive, and that could make for an uncomfortable work environment.

SAMPLE CONFIDENTIALITY AGREEMENT

AGREEMENT by and between

(Company) and   , (Undersigned),

Whereas, the Company agrees to allow the Undersigned access to certain confidential information, trade secrets, or proprietary information relating to the affairs of the Company only for purposes of:

, and

Whereas, the Undersigned and its agents, attorneys, accountants or advisors may review, examine, inspect, have access to or obtain such information only for the purposes described above, and to otherwise hold such disclosed information confidential pursuant to the terms of this agreement

BE IT ACKNOWLEDGED, that the Company has or shall furnish to the Undersigned certain confidential information, described on the attached list, and Company may further allow the Undersigned the right to inspect the business of the Company and/or interview suppliers, customers, employees or representatives of the Company, only on the following conditions:

1.   The Undersigned agrees to hold all disclosed confidential or proprietary information or trade secrets ("information") in trust and confidence and agrees that it shall be used only for the contemplated purpose, and shall not be used for any other purpose nor disclosed to any third party without written consent of Company.

2.   No copies or abstracts will be made or retained of any written information supplied. Upon demand by the Company, all information, including written notes, photographs, or memoranda shall be returned to the Company.

3.   The disclosed information shall not be disclosed to any employee, consultant or third party unless said party agrees to execute and be bound by the terms of this agreement.

4.   It is understood that the Undersigned shall have no obligation to hold confidential with respect to any information known by the Undersigned or generally known within the industry prior to date of this agreement, or that shall become common knowledge within the industry thereafter as said information shall not be deemed protected under this agreement.

5.   The Undersigned acknowledges the information disclosed herein constitutes proprietary and trade secrets and in the event of unlawful use or wrongful disclosure, the Company shall be entitled to injunctive relief as a cumulative and not necessarily successive remedy without need to post bond.

6.   This agreement shall be binding upon and inure to the benefit of the parties, their successors, assigns and personal representatives.

Special provisions:

Signed under seal this   day of   , 19   .

Signed in the presence of:

_____   _____

_____   _____

Sample Confidentiality Agreement, check with your legal counsel for one which specifically fits your needs.

SAMPLE NON-COMPETITION AGREEMENT

FOR VALUE RECEIVED and other good consideration, the undersigned

jointly and severally covenant and agree not to compete with the business of

located at

("Company") and its lawful successors and
assigns, pursuant to the terms hereof.

The term "not compete" as used herein shall mean that the undersigned shall not directly or indirectly engage in a business or other activity generally described as:

notwithstanding whether said participation be as an owner, officer, director, employee, agent, consultant, partner or stockholder (except as a passive stockholder in a publicly owned company).

This covenant not to compete shall extend only for a radius of   miles from the present location of the Company at   , and shall remain in full force and effect for   years from date hereof whereupon it shall terminate.

In the event of any breach, the Company shall be entitled to full injunctive relief without need to post bond, which rights shall be cumulative with and not necessarily successive or exclusive of any other legal rights.

This Agreement shall be binding upon and inure to the benefit of the parties, their successors, assigns and personal representatives.

Upon breach the undersigned shall be responsible for all reasonable attorneys fees and costs incurred in the enforcement of this agreement.

Special provisions:

Signed under seal this   day of   , 19   .

Signed in the presence of:

_____   _____

_____   _____

Acknowledged by (Company)

_____

Sample Non-competition Agreement, check with your legal counsel for one which specifically fits your needs.

❦ **Review and Summary** ❦

You should now have a very good idea of what it means to negotiate: finding out what the physician wants, putting together
your wants and needs, and then coming to a mutual understanding. The job offer and acceptance is not based only on an hourly
wage; it is the sum of other parts, including benefits, the time
you spend working, and how close is the job description to what
you wanted to be doing in a medical practice.

There is no exact formula for determining the amount of
revenue that adding esthetic services could bring into the practice. By breaking down various treatment costs, the productivity
of a one-hour treatment will give the physician and esthetician a
good idea of the profitability of adding esthetic services. If you
are a seasoned esthetician you know or found out quickly that
for the next forty years you will only be able to see forty patients
a week if you see one-hour patients. Therefore, you realize that
the profit earned working in a medical practice or salon environment is in product sales. This is an aspect that the physician may
not understand. Educating the physician on the profitability of
product sales may be entirely up to the esthetician.

A positive attitude is a plus while negotiating the employment agreement and turning the negotiation into a win-win situation. Always keep in mind that the additional benefits may
bring your employment package into a more favorable light.
Here I am talking about health insurance. Health insurance can
cost up to 300 dollars per month, especially if family is involved.
The benefit of a 401K Plan or profit sharing can go a long way
toward building a retirement nest egg. Another factor that can be
negotiated into the employment offer is vacation time. If you
have small children it would be to your advantage to have four
to six weeks. If it is necessary for you to bring down your hourly
wage in order to get four to six weeks vacation to spend quality
time with your children, it is a trade-off that should be looked at
as a positive benefit.

The trade-offs of working as an independent contractor or as
an employee should have become obvious.

The esthetician's job description is something that will
change from practice to practice. The example used in this chapter is meant to be used as a guide. However, it may vary depending on the area of medical specialty. It is a good idea to have a

copy of the esthetician's job description clearly outlined and signed before accepting the entire employment package. If you do not have a written job description it will be difficult later on when discussing what the physician expected of you.

In the sample employment agreement, the terms of employment, your job description, and what you expect from the employer were discussed. The agreement also completely outlines the compensation package: performance bonus, vacation days, and additional benefits. The confidentiality and non-solicitation of patients is very important while working in a medical practice.

Finally, medicine is often a tense occupation. Some people remain calm and courteous even under the most trying circumstances; others become short-tempered and impolite. Be sensitive to the style the physician maintains in moments of relaxation, during routine office procedures, when confronted with emergencies, when talking to pleasant patients, and when dealing with difficult ones. This is the person you'll be working with day in and day out, possibly for years. If you're comfortable together, this could be a great position; if not, it could be very difficult and unpleasant for both of you.

Ask yourself the following questions:

- Do you feel comfortable discussing issues with the physician?

- Is there a clear line of communication between you and the physician?

- Do you feel that you can discuss patient issues with the physician?

- Does the physician seem open to new ideas and respect your opinions?

- Do you feel the the physician has the patience to teach you the additional information you will need to know in order to be a valuable member of the health care team?

- Have you taken the time to calculate approximately how much additional income you will contribute to the physician's practice?

- Have you carefully considered the salary you would need to pay for your expenses?

- What do you need beyond salary, such as additional benefits, including health insurance, retirement plans, and tuition reimbursement?

- Do you know the practice's policy on overtime, sick leave, and vacations?

- Do you understand the pros and cons of working as a private contractor?

- Are your proposed duties and responsibilities clear to you?

- Have you thought about the implications of signing a non-compete clause?

Chapter Six

Insurance
and
Liability Issues

In this chapter you will learn:

- ■ how to protect yourself from a lawsuit

- ■ what types of insurance you'll need whether you work as an independent contractor or as an employee of a physician

- ■ how the details of your state-issued esthetic license may affect the kind of insurance coverage you may need

- ■ how to reduce your liability by obtaining an informed consent

Though you hope you never use it, you absolutely need insurance. I'm not talking about your health insurance or life insurance; important as they are, you can live without them. But professional liability insurance isn't an option, it's a necessity. We live in an especially litigious society, where the chances of being sued are probably greater than anywhere else on earth. And recent studies suggest that the procedures over which patients are most likely to sue are not the unusual ones, but the procedures that are performed by physicians every day, including suits for failing to perform a procedure, which is to say, for performing no procedure at all!

Take Cover—Insurance for Estheticians in a Medical Setting

As an esthetician, you perform services every day that leave you vulnerable to being sued by patients who are actually harmed or who believe they've been harmed by something you've done to them, something you've failed to do, or by a product you've used, sold, or recommended. This is true if you work in a salon, but the risks may be a little different for estheticians working in a medical practice, especially today. Patients often take a somewhat adversarial stance when they go to a physician, which helps explain the explosion in medical malpractice suits in recent years. Of course, most patients you'll see won't even think of suing, and to an extent, the press has probably exaggerated the problem of frivolous lawsuits and contentious patients, but no matter how small the risk, neither you nor the physician you work with can afford to take it. Hence, insurance is needed, which may be defined as trading a potentially large but uncertain loss for a small but certain cost.

When It Comes to Insurance, You Must Get Professional Advice

I'm going to cover two related areas, limiting your liability (reducing the risk that you or the physician you work for could be sued by something you do or fail to do) and insuring yourself against any claims that might arise if you are in fact sued. But before I go any further, I must tell you that insurance is one area that you can't afford to leave to amateurs, and in this area, I am an amateur. I can outline the steps you should take to manage the risk of being sued, and I can tell you in a general way about the kinds of insurance available, but insurance law is very specific and it varies from state to state. The only way to be sure you have the coverage you need is to consult an insurance professional, specifically an insurance agent who specializes in insuring estheticians and who is experienced in the issues involved when estheticians work in a medical setting.

If you've been working in a salon, whether you've been an employee or independent contractor, you probably have insurance coverage. (If you don't, you've been taking an enormous risk.) Your present insurance agent is a good place to start when researching the coverage you'll need when you move to a medical setting, but don't be shy about asking the agent if he or she knows the specific requirements of insuring estheticians working in medical settings. If the agent is unsure of what's involved, and if the agent is reputable, the agent will make the necessary calls and do the research needed to find out. Or the agent may suggest you call someone more expert in this specific field. Whatever you do, make sure the advice you're getting is based on fact, not conjecture. When you're actually sued is no time to find out that the policy you've been relying on won't really protect you. The rule, as always, is that an ounce of prevention is worth a pound (in the case of inflated jury awards, a ton) of cure.

Because the field is so new, and because insurance law varies from state to state, it's difficult to talk in general terms about what insurance you need and how to obtain it. Generally, you'll need to be covered under the physician's liability policy, and since those policies don't necessarily automatically cover people working in the office, you'll have to be specifically added to the policy. For the most part, companies don't cover estheticians specifically; rather, you'll be listed as a medical assistant. And while your own coverage may protect you from procedures you routinely perform in a salon, it may not cover you for procedures you do in a physician's office, especially if you perform procedures outside of those your state license covers. For instance, the most controversial treatment is the application of chemical exfoliating agents. Each state cosmetology board had its own definition of what is considered safe practice of applying chemical agents to the face of a client/patient.

According to the California Board of Barbering and Cosmetology, "...a chemical exfoliation is a process by which layers of facial skin are removed with commercially available products. Skin peel acids are applied to the face for a few minutes a day over several days. The skin reddens like a sunburn, darkens, and peels away, revealing a layer of sensitive, new skin. Recovery time varies from days to weeks or even longer depending on the depth of the peel."

According to the Nevada State Board of Cosmetology, "...[they] mandated a policy that products using the terminology PEEL and are used for EXFOLIATION only, can continue to be utilized, however an ingredients list as well as how the product is being used must be submitted to the Board so that this information may be kept in record."

Should you maintain the insurance you had before you started working in a medical office? Generally speaking, yes. In fact, in some cases, the physician's insurance company will require that you maintain your own policy in order to be added to the physician's liability package. Even when you're not required to keep it, it's generally a good idea to maintain the policy you had; it is relatively inexpensive, and it offers additional protection. And since the physician's liability insurance covers you only for procedures you do in the physician's office, if you work outside of the office, you'll need to have your own coverage.

Independent Contractors

This information about insurance pertains to estheticians who work as employees in a medical office; it does not refer to estheticians working as independent contractors or who rent space in a physician's practice. Independent contractors have entirely different insurance needs; they generally must maintain much more extensive liability insurance, including so-called "slip and fall" coverage to protect them from liability if someone has an accident in the space they rent, as well as insurance against theft of equipment, business interruption, etc. I don't recommend that estheticians work as independent contractors or rent space in a medical practice, and the insurance issue is only one reason. If, however, this is what you decide to do, make sure you discuss your needs very carefully with an insurance agent who is familiar with esthetic practices in medical settings.

Heading Trouble Off Before It Starts—Reducing Risk

Prevention is most important to insure yourself against being sued. The first line of defense is making sure that you've done everything you can to reduce as much as possible the possibility of being sued, which is another way of saying reducing your liability. Reducing liability—risk management, in insurance-company jargon—is what we do when we shovel our sidewalks so people won't slip on them, or when we pick up stray toys so visitors won't fall in our homes. And just as there are specific things that should be done to limit liability as homeowners, hosts, or temporary employers of repairmen, there are specific things that can and should be done to limit liability in a medical office.

While the physician is ultimately responsible for what happens (or doesn't happen) in the medical office, you should be aware of certain standard practices that are designed to minimize liability. Actual implementation of these practices may be up to the physician, but if you are aware of something that should be done to reduce risk that's being neglected, you should immediately bring it to the physician's attention. While the physician is the head of the medical team, as a member of that team, you should do your part to make sure that it functions at all times as well as it can.

Going by the Rules

At the heart of any risk-reduction program is a set of standard operating procedures that have been designed to limit liability. Often referred to as "protocols," they act as constant guidelines, assuring that you and the rest of the office practice according to a given set of standards. The crucial thing about establishing protocols is that they take the guesswork out of deciding what to do or how to act in any of the situations covered. Protocols cover just about everything that goes on in a medical practice, from how to answer the phone and schedule appointments to how to sterilize which instruments.

If the entire office operates strictly according to the established protocols, the risk of anyone doing anything that will increase the office's liability is minimized. The rules are useless, of course, if they aren't stated in writing and if they aren't clearly understood and followed at all times by everyone in the office. This is why it is so important for you to ask to see and study the written protocols in the office before you actually do any work there. Knowing the rules protects you and the physician for whom you'll be working.

Because these protocols vary from office to office, it is difficult to go into detail about them, but certain underlying principles will prevail in any medical setting. Some of the more common ones are discussed below.

Informed Consent

Obtaining the patient's **informed consent** for any treatment he or she receives is obviously essential in limiting liability if anything goes wrong. A patient who suffers an irritation or a burn from a chemical agent applied to the skin, who can show that no one ever told him this was a possibility, is in a strong position to sue. That's not to say the patient will win the suit, but failing to obtain the "informed consent" for the procedure definitely increases the possibility that the patient will recover some monetary award, and if you performed the procedure, you as well as the physician could be named as a defendant.

Of course limiting liability isn't the only reason to obtain informed consent. There's clearly a moral responsibility to explain the possible adverse effects of treatments and procedures. And there are important medical benefits as well. Patients who understand the nature of their ailment and the nature of the proposed treatment or cosmetic procedure are less likely to be apprehensive, and reducing anxiety not only makes the patient (and the practitioner) more comfortable, it can actually improve the results. In addition, patients who understand the procedure or treatment are more likely to comply with follow-up or home care.

The physician bears the ultimate responsibility for obtaining informed consent from the patient, but the physician may well delegate some of the responsibility to others. In some practices, the physician explains all the procedures to the patient and obtains written consent beforehand. In others, the physician explains only his or her procedures, and leaves to staff members the responsibility to explain and obtain consent for the procedures the staff will handle themselves. The physician is still responsible for making sure the patient understands the procedure and its possible adverse effects, but the actual interview with the patient and the obtaining of the written consent may be left to the esthetician. As long as you follow the prescribed format in both your discussions and in the written consent form the patient signs, you're probably safe. Just make sure you don't cut any corners, rushing through your explanation or even skipping the actual form and letting the patient receive the treatment before you've received the signed consent.

Obtaining informed consent is a two-part process; discussion always precedes the actual written form. During the discussion, the physician or whoever is responsible for obtaining consent

Sample Consent Form

I hereby consent to and authorize Dr._____and/or his assistants to perform the procedure of _____upon myself.

I fully understand the necessity and/or elective reasoning of this procedure, which has been explained to me by Dr._____and/or his assistants.

As with any procedure, I also understand that there are certain risks involved. These include the possibility of further treatment of the treated sites, hypertrophic and/or keloid scarring, and hyper- or hypopigmentation of the skin.

As far as my treatment course, I understand that there is a chance of swelling, bruising, and/or some mild and/or moderate discomfort which are all normal occurrences of this procedure.

I agree to follow to the best of my ability all postoperative instruction given to me by Dr._____and/or his assistant. I understand that instruction and/or medication involved are for the best healing and cosmesis of the areas treated.

I have also, to the best of my knowledge, given an accurate account of my past medical history, including all known allergies, to Dr._____ and/or his assistant and fully understand the information above.

Date_____

Patient's Signature _____

Physician's Signature _____

Witness _____

Sample Consent Form, check with your legal counsel for one which specifically fits your needs.

Sample Procedure Consent Form for Micropigmentation

Name _____Address _____

City _____ State _____ Zip _____

Phone Home (   ) _____ Work (   ) _____

Referred by _____ Procedure_____

Do you take Zovirax?	No	Yes
Do you wear contact lenses?	No	Yes
Do you have any kind of heart trouble?	No	Yes
Are you a diabetic?	No	Yes
Are you taking recreational drugs?	No	Yes
Are you able to take Benadryl?	No	Yes
Are you allergic to novocaine?	No	Yes
Do you get fever blisters/cold sores?	No	Yes
Have you ever tested positive for HIV?	No	Yes
Are you presently taking any medication?	No	Yes

List: _____

Fees discussed _____ Deposit _____ Balance _____
I fully understand that a consultation fee of $50.00 will be deducted from my deposit in the event of cancellation of said procedure. The entire staff is dedicated to client satisfaction. We employ a no-refund policy, and I am aware of this. x _____ Date
_____

I absolutely understand that this procedure is a process and subsequent visits are necessary in order to achieve desired results. Subsequent visits are subject to $100/$300 charge depending upon the amount of work needed. It is understood that I have received a patch test prior to application, which releases _____ and assistants from any liability related to any allergic or other reaction to applied pigments.(Pigment contents: iron oxide, alcohol, distilled water, glycerine) I acknowledge that no guarantees have been made to me concerning the results of this procedure. For the purpose of documentation, I also consent to the taking of before-and-after photographs of said procedure, which may or may not be used by _____. I have read the above and had explained to me and fully understand this consent and procedure form: That the explanations therein referred to were made and I accept full responsibility for these or any other complications that may arise from results during or following the cosmetic procedure(s) which is to be performed at my request according to this consent and procedure form. x _____ Date _____

_____

Patient Signature

_____

Physician Signature

_____

Witness Signature

Sample Procedure Consent Form, check with your legal counsel for one which specifically fits your needs.

explains the nature of the patient's problem or condition; the nature of the proposed treatment and what the treatment is designed to accomplish; the benefits of this treatment or procedure; the risks and alternatives to it; and, in some cases, the risks of no treatment, which may include the exacerbation of a medical condition or adverse effects of an esthetic problem. The important thing is that the explanation be geared to the patient's understanding and that the patient have a chance to ask any questions. Stick to clear terms and avoid jargon. On the other hand, don't talk down to your patient. Above all, be honest. If there will be a moderate amount of pain or discomfort, don't lie about it. The worst thing about medical procedures for many patients is not the actual discomfort involved but the fear of not knowing what will happen.

Exactly what is "informed consent"? I'm not a lawyer, and the case law, the results of actual trials in this area, is not clear and varies from state to state. Suffice it to say that patients who are not themselves expert in the procedures they're consenting to are not expected to have an expert's knowledge of the possible adverse effects associated with those procedures. How much do you have to explain? Do you have to mention that one patient in a million may experience a certain side effect? One in ten thousand? One in a hundred? Do you have to go into details about what could go wrong but probably won't?

Since there are no definite rules about what patients need to know, you're safe if you rely on common sense. You should explain what a reasonable person would want to know in order to decide whether or not to have a certain treatment or procedure. If it is extremely unlikely that the patient will experience a certain adverse effect, you're probably safe not going into it. However, with a procedure like a chemical exfoliation, despite the general safety of the procedure, there is a real risk that a patient might experience discomfort, a mild burn, or an allergic reaction. You should definitely make sure the patient understands what these risks are and how likely he or she is to experience them.

Whatever the procedure, it is your responsibility to explain it, make sure the patient understands what you've said, and make sure you obtain a written consent form. The only exceptions are if the physician has already obtained a written consent that covers the treatment or procedure that you're going to give.

Triage

You've no doubt seen it in war movies or on TV hospital dramas, dozens of incoming casualties, stretchers being rushed through swinging doors into the emergency room, some to be treated immediately or rushed to the operating room, others to be put on the side with a few words of comfort and assurance. What you're watching is **triage**, a word derived from a French word that means to sort or sift. In medical terms, triage is the process of assigning to a patient in need of care a level of urgency for that care. A patient who presents at the emergency room with a gunshot wound to the abdomen obviously is in more urgent need of care than a young adult who comes in with what appears to be a case of the flu. The gunshot wound will be taken care of immediately, with all available resources. The patient with the flu will be asked to wait until a physician or nurse is available to assess his needs.

You're not going to work in an emergency room, but you will be faced with analogous situations, and in some cases, you may even have to judge between patients who are seriously ill or in crisis and those who can wait until the physician can conveniently see them. If you fail to recognize the urgency of a patient's complaint and you fail to act appropriately, you and the practice could become liable for damages.

The person primarily responsible for making sure that patients who have a genuine medical emergency are seen quickly is the physician. You are not expected to be a diagnostician, after all, but the practice as a whole is expected to have established clear triage guidelines, clear protocols for handling telephone calls and walk-in patients. Everyone who has direct contact with patients, whether in person or on the phone, is expected to know these guidelines and to follow them scrupulously.

A number of things are covered by the triage protocols, including:

■ the guidelines for determining which patients need immediate appointments with the physician and which can wait until the next available opening;

■ which prescriptions can be renewed by phone by an assigned assistant and which need the physician's personal attention (generally speaking only the physician will authorize or renew prescriptions for narcotics and antibiotics, among other drugs);

■ which calls need to be answered immediately by the physician, which can be returned later, and which can be handled by you or a nurse.

In addition to limiting liability, following accepted, established guidelines is the best way to assure that patients who really need to be seen or who need advice right away are properly taken care of. It guarantees that emergencies receive priority, and that can make the difference between a procedure that's successful and one that fails, and in some cases, it may even make the difference between life and death.

A Matter of Privacy

One of the most important tenets of the patient-physician relationship is that the patient has the right to expect that everything said to the physician, everything the physician says, the details of the diagnosis and treatment, and all records will remain confidential unless the patient gives explicit written permission to share them with another party. As a member of the physician's staff and as someone who has access to confidential information about patients—even the fact that someone is a physician's patient—you are bound by the same strict rules about **patient confidentiality.** Failure to keep information confidential can cause a patient great pain and can be grounds for a successful lawsuit.

Under no circumstances should you ever reveal anything about a patient to anyone on the phone or in person without the express permission of the physician. Except under certain very limited legal circumstances, generally defined by a court order, no information about a patient, including patient records, can be released to anyone without first obtaining a signed release form from the patient. Neither employers nor insurance companies, neither family members nor friends, have any right to information about a patient, unless written consent is given. The rule is simple: refer anyone who wants such information to the physician. Sometimes an impatient employer or insurance company or a deeply concerned spouse or family member may insist that you reveal something about a patient. Don't. Ever.

Respecting a patient's privacy goes beyond knowingly releasing information about the patient. It extends to making sure that patient records are stored carefully in an area where they won't be accessible to other patients or people in the office who are not directly involved with patient care or have some other valid reason for access to them. It also means that you will never let others overhear phone conversations with the patient or conversations between you and the physician about the patient or the patient's care. And respecting patient privacy goes beyond the office. You must be careful to avoid discussing patients with your friends or family members. Don't give in to the temptation to reveal that a well-known person was in the office, and don't think that simply not revealing a patient's name gives you the right to talk about the patient. Patients have a right to believe that their privacy will be absolutely protected. You have an absolute responsibility to see that it is.

Most of what we've said about limiting liability and protecting yourself against lawsuits is common sense. By following written protocols, by respecting the absolute right to privacy that every patient enjoys, and by acting in a mature, responsible way, you will limit the risk that you or the practice will be held responsible for any damages. You'll protect your economic health and, just as important, your peace of mind.

ϒ Review and Summary ϒ

Talking about insurance and the liability issues of the esthetician working in a medical practice is difficult. The area of insurance for estheticians in a medical setting is so new that many gray areas need to be addressed by both the physician and the esthetician. Issues such as whether the esthetician works as an independent contractor or an employee can imply many things with reference to liability. Also, the esthetician's license may affect the insurance coverage. In some states estheticians working in medical practices cannot call themselves estheticians, so therefore how would the physician insure?

Both the esthetician and physician need to be aware of these issues and plan on how to reduce their liability. Obtaining informed consent is one way to do that. I generally recommend that estheticians maintain their own malpractice or liability insurance and that the physician obtain a written letter from his/her medical malpractice carrier stating that they will cover the esthetician when they do procedures in the physician's office, stipulating whether or not the physician needs to be on the premises while the procedure is being performed. There are certainly different insurance needs, and each liability carrier will address it in their own way. While doing research for this book I contacted six different medical malpractice insurance carriers and was given six different answers!

Following strict protocols and consistently used guidelines may help to assure that the esthetician and physician avoid a lawsuit. The patient-physician relationship is one of utmost privacy, and the details of their diagnosis and treatment and all medical records are deemed confidential. Therefore, the esthetician working in a medical practice must become familiar with matters of privacy and the strict rules that bind the physician-patient relationship. Failure to keep this information confidential is certainly grounds for a lawsuit.

Most of what I have said about limiting liability and protecting yourself from lawsuits is common sense. By following written protocols, by respecting the absolute right to privacy that every patient enjoys, and by acting in a mature, responsible way, the physician and the esthetician can limit the risk for the practice. Protecting your economic health is just as important as your peace of mind.

Ask yourself the following questions:

- Do you know the practice's policy on patient confidentiality as it pertains to their medical records?

- What can you do to protect yourself from incurring a liability suit while performing esthetic procedures?

- Are you carrying sufficient liability insurance for the types of procedures that you will be performing in the physician's practice?

- Do you know exactly how well (or poorly) the physician's insurance protects you?

Chapter Seven

Practice Administration

Sarah Wiskerchen

In this chapter you will learn:

- ■ practice administration such as telephone communication
- ■ how to determine referral trends in your esthetic practice
- ■ the process of balancing at the end of the day
- ■ important points of successful patient scheduling

Office Policies and Procedures

An esthetic practice uniquely combines features of a general medical practice in providing various skin-care services and products that complement the surgical procedures performed by a physician. This combination offers physicians and estheticians the opportunity to provide a spectrum of complementary services to patients, which are designed to improve the appearance and self-image of the patients.

The creation and use of consistent policies and procedures in the esthetic practice enables physicians, estheticians, and their staff to provide a congruous environment to patients. Continuous training regarding the procedures and services provided, a patient service focus, and streamlined operational systems all contribute to this environment.

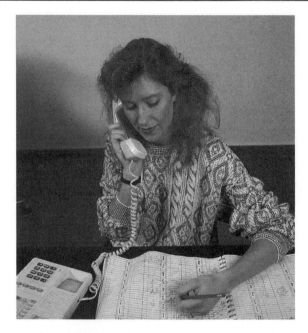

The first telephone contact is crucial in retaining a patient's attention and interest.

Making the Connection—Telephone Communication in Action

While the saying "first impressions make the difference" may seem overused and outdated, it continues to hold true in service industries of all types. In a market where plastic surgeons, dermatologists, and facial plastic surgeons are competing with one another, making the most of that first impression is essential.

While your traditional media marketing efforts may serve as the initial contact point for many of your patients, their first telephone interaction with your practice will serve as a crucial "moment of truth" when it comes to retaining the patient's attention and interest. To make the most of the initial contact, the receptionist should:

■ Answer the telephone promptly—within three rings.

Think of your frustration when phoning a business where the phone is answered on the eighth or tenth ring, or you are immediately placed on hold. Monitor your telephone call volume for busy signals and holding patterns, and query patients about their ability to reach your facility. "Christmas tree" phone lines are a warning signal that your system is at maximum capacity—you may need additional lines or staff to support them. Don't allow that potential patient to hang up and call another practice!

■ Put a smile in his or her voice.

Smiling helps the speaker place more enthusiasm in his or her voice, and helps to put the potential patient at ease. Many customer-focused businesses place a small mirror at eye level near the telephone as a reminder for staff to maintain a smile even when patients are not physically present.

■ Be well-versed in the services and products you provide.

Limiting staff access to information and training will only handicap their efforts to provide the customer service you wish to encourage. Staff members should participate in regular in-house training sessions that review the features of the various services and products you provide, and the advantages you offer over other practices. The support staff provide the link to the patient and are a reflection of the care you as the esthetician will provide. The staff should be equipped to achieve success in contributing to your skin-care efforts.

Do not wait until the patient's visit to differentiate your practice from the competition. The patient may be contacting a number of providers—make sure you are the one that leaves a lasting, positive impression.

■ Offer flexible scheduling options.

Most potential customers today lead busy life-styles. Consider the times of greatest patient need as you establish office hours. Many medical practices today offer evening hours to serve working patients who have trouble keeping daytime appointments. Scheduling contributes to the level of patient satisfaction at a very basic level—accommodating the patient's timing needs will allow them to relax and make the most of the visit.

■ Provide written information upon request.

Many potential patients need time to consider the options available before buying. Volunteer to send patient information materials, such as a practice brochure or a list of services, even if they do not immediately schedule an appointment. Be sure to include a description of your financial policies and your guidelines regarding insurance coverage. (Many patients mistakenly believe that skin-care services are covered by insurances. While this may be true in limited situations, the practice is not obligated to understand each individual's policy limits.) Consider how you can use personal fax or e-mail communications to speed up the contact process, keeping in mind the patient's preferences regarding confidentiality. Add the potential patient's name to your marketing lists for future use.

Telephone Do's and Don'ts

Don't Say:

She's all booked up. She can't see you until _____.

Say:

(Name) is scheduled at that time, but she can see you at _____.

I'm sorry, I can't fit you in today.

It's a shame you weren't able to call earlier, but (Name) can see you tomorrow.

(Name) is running late.

(Name) has an interrupted schedule.

Remind.

Confirm, verify.

Cancellation.

Change in schedule.

Recall.

Follow-up visit or preventive program.

She's an "old" patient of (Name).

Former patient, continuing patient, established patient.

You misunderstood.

There was a misunderstanding.

Are you a patient here?

When did we last see you?

What do you want?

How may I help you?

All patients pay cash.

We appreciate your payment at the time of the visit. We do accept cash, checks, and major credit cards.

I know.

I understand.

Free.

Complimentary.

Telephone Tracking

Understanding how patients learned about your services is key to the future development of your marketing plan. The evaluation of your efforts begins with good record keeping, beginning when the potential patient contacts the practice. Educate staff on the importance of accurate tracking records, and instruct the receptionist to obtain as much information as possible during the first phone call.

This form should be completed by the receptionist at the time the potential patient calls, even if no visit is scheduled at that time.

Sample Telephone Tracking Form

Date/Time Taken: _____

Patient Name: _____

Mailing Address: _____

Phone Numbers: Home (   ) _____

                   Work (   ) _____

Initial Interest: _____

_____

Referred By: _____

Information Sent: _____

Prices Quoted: _____

Date of Visit: _____

Taken By: _____

This card should be completed by the patient at the first visit. It allows you to review the reasons the patient may have chosen to see you. The receptionist should add the patient's name and the services and products purchased after the visit.

This information should be collated each quarter to determine what referral trends may be affecting the practice.

How Did You Learn About Skin Care Associates?

Please circle all statements that apply:

1. My friend, _____ told me about _____

2. My physician, _____ told me about _____

3. Your location is convenient to my home or office.

4. I noticed your yellow pages ad.

5. I noticed your newspaper ad in_____

6. I heard your radio ad on station _____

7. I heard _____ speak at the educational seminar on _____

8. I read your newsletter.

9. Other_____

Reception Services—The Process

Once the patient has scheduled an appointment and arrived in the office, the need for service focus and attention continues. The following ideas focus on the reception area process, and some key interactions that take place between office staff and the patient.

1. Establish a patient-friendly environment.

   First, consider the physical space you have allocated for esthetic services. Does the esthetic area share a reception area with other practice patients? Think about the comfort level of seating and lighting, and the types of reading material you have provided for patients. You may wish to provide a combination of materials that describe

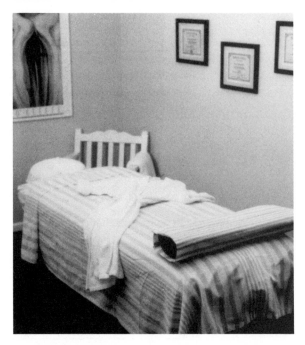

Be sure to create a "patient-friendly" environment for esthetic services.

both surgical and skin-care services. Pay close attention to the way voices carry through the office. If conversations in the patient care area can be overheard, you may need to include some soft background music to mask the noise and prevent information from being overheard. Be sure to provide display space for your skin-care products, especially cosmetics. Often patients will ask to test colors and textures even before they have participated in the skin-care visit.

2. Greet the patient with genuine warmth and attention.

Continue the communication style that originated during the telephone contact with the patient. Make sure the staff also treats the patients in the office with genuine warmth and enthusiasm. Many patients prefer to be greeted by name, rather than with a simple nod or glance. Once the patient arrives, the staff should be instructed to gather all pertinent demographic information, and request the patient to complete the "Where

Did You Learn About Us" information card. This is another opportunity for the staff to answer any questions the patients may have, and to explain financial policies for the practice. Once the receptionist has all the information needed, the patient should be invited to take a seat until the appointment time.

3. Following the skin-care visit.

After the esthetician has provided the scheduled skin-care service, the patient can be escorted back to the reception area. As noted previously, by this time the patient should have had the opportunity to address all product and service questions with the esthetician. The esthetician should provide the receptionist with an esthetic encounter form, which includes all skin-care services and products. The esthetician will have circled all services provided, as well as products the patient wishes to purchase. The esthetician should also indicate how soon the patient is advised to return for follow-up. Using the encounter form, the cashier can then obtain payment for the services rendered and products requested, fill the patient's product order, and schedule the appropriate follow-up visit for the patient. Be sure to provide a reminder card that notes the next visit date, and remind the patient that a staff member will phone to remind them within three days of the visit. Take this face-to-face opportunity to remind the patient of your cancellation policy.

4. Balancing the day.

Just as audit controls are necessary in a traditional medical practice, they are required in the esthetic practice setting. The following steps should be completed to ensure that all receipts for services match money collected by the staff.

Once the last patient has left for the day, do the following:

■ Complete posting (or logging) of payments and charges from services provided during the day and products purchased. Total all services and corresponding payments received.

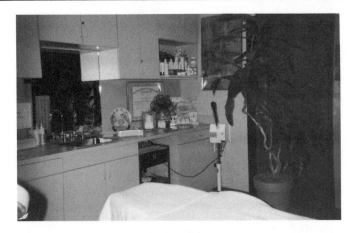

Esthetic treatment room

■ Account for any encounter forms not yet entered into the computer system or logged manually. Once they are located and closed out, enter the numbers of all encounter forms at the top of the Daily Close Form.

■ Complete the Daily Close Form (See sample Daily Close Form, page 143.) Follow these steps and be sure to save your adding machine tape:

1. Total all reception cash received.

2. Total all reception checks received.

3. Total all charge card receipts.

4. Enter the total of these on Line 4.

5. Compare these totals with the totals of services and products provided. If the totals match, enter the total from Line 4 in the "total" space on Line 5. If the totals do not match, you must go through and account for the differential.

■ Make copies of all checks received. Make sure you have stamped all checks for deposit. Prepare a deposit ticket and deliver it to the office manager, along with appropriate stamped checks, credit card vouchers, and cash.

■ Fasten together the check copies, Daily Close Form, all encounter forms, and the adding machine tape that shows your work, and give them to the office manager.

Sample Daily Close Form

Accounting date: _____

Prepared by (initial after your portion is complete): _____

Encounter forms from _____ through _____

Reception Services

1. Over-the-counter cash $ _____

2. Over-the-counter checks $ _____

3. VISA/Mastercard/Discover $ _____

4. Total: Lines 1 + 2 + 3 $ _____

5. Report total (on deposit slip report) $ _____

6. Over/Under (Lines 4 and 5) $ _____

When lines 4 and 5 balance, the day is balanced.

Plus Any Additional Payments (itemize)

_____ $ _____

_____ $ _____

_____ $ _____

_____ $ _____

_____ $ _____

Total To Deposit $ _____

Patient Records—The Importance of Documentation

As a complement to a medical/surgical practice, the esthetician is required to document the services provided as part of the patient's medical record. This provides the physician with a clear picture of the patient's spectrum of care, and also provides the esthetician with an understanding of the medical plan recommended by the physician. If the patient is not a regular patient of the dermatologist or surgeon, establish a plan for those records that will be consistent with all others in the practice.

If the practice does integrate medical and esthetic services completely, the esthetic staff will need to participate in regular documentation training. The following "Principles of Documentation" addresses those items that must be included in a medical record, whether by the physician or esthetician.

Principles of Documentation

1. The medical record should be complete and legible.

2. The documentation of each patient encounter should include: the date, the reason for the encounter, appropriate history and physical exam; review of ancillary test results, where appropriate; assessment; and plan for care.

3. Past and present diagnoses should be accessible to the treating and/or consulting physician.

4. Relevant health risk factors should be identified.

5. The patient's progress, including response to treatment, change in treatment, change in diagnosis, and patient noncompliance, should be documented.

6. The written plan for care should include, when appropriate: treatments and medications, specifying frequency and dosage; any referrals and consultations; patient/family education; and specific instructions for follow-up.

7. The documentation should support the intensity of the patient evaluation and/or the treatment, including thought processes and the complexity of medical decision-making.

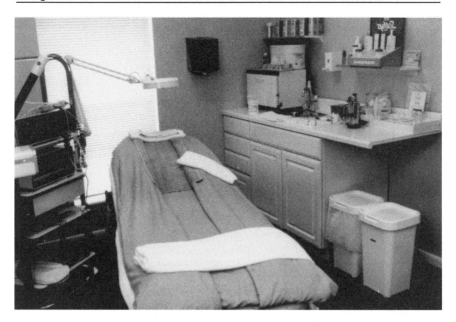

Time intervals for appointments should include time for turning over the treatment room for the next patient visit.

    8. All entries to the medical record should be dated and authenticated.

For best results in your documentation efforts, look into the opportunity to dictate and transcribe your notes for the medical record. This helps you to meet the legibility requirement. The record should also include a roster of skin-care products purchased and the patient's comments and feedback following their use.

Patient Scheduling

As noted previously, patient scheduling should be arranged in a patient-focused manner. At the same time, productivity for the esthetician and physician is a vital concern.

As a first step, decide what time intervals are required for the services you will provide. Additionally, consider the time needed to turn the room over for the next patient visit. The esthetician will need to concentrate on patient education regarding products and other services while they remain in the room with the patient. This will minimize delays for the esthetician when meeting the schedule for the next patient.

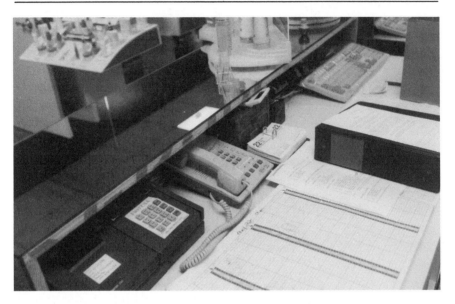

Successful scheduling includes calling patients two days in advance to remind them about appointments.

Once you have established a steady patient stream for esthetic skin-care services, be sure to implement a waiting list for patients who may be interested in moving their appointment to an earlier time. Should a cancellation occur, these patients can be contacted immediately, possibly avoiding inefficient down time in the schedule.

Many practices enforce a cancellation policy whereby twenty-four hour notice is required. Otherwise, a fee will be assessed to the patient. Ideally, you should be able to schedule follow-up visits several months beyond the current date—do not be held hostage by short-term decision-making for vacations and time off. Encourage the patient to schedule two to three months of visits at once to ensure the time is available for them.

Important Points of Successful Scheduling

1. Calling to remind patients of appointments two days in advance.

2. Notifying patients whenever they call to schedule or change appointments of twenty-four-hour **notice of cancellation policy** to avoid last minute schedule openings.

February Day 26 Date

	1 Sally	2 Joan	3
8 00 15 30 45			
9 00 15 30 45			Take name, H & W Telephone #s
10 00 15 30 45			
11 00 15 30 45			
12 00 15 30 45			
1 00 15 30 45			
2 00 15 30 45	LUNCH		
3 00 15 30 45			
4 00 15 30 45			
5 00 15 30 45			
6 00 15 30 45			
7 00 15 30 45			

3. Ask new patients to arrive fifteen minutes before appointment time in order to fill out new patient information.

4. Appointment booking codes will help to keep the book organized and easy to do follow-up.

NP   New Patient

CX   Cancellation

B   Booked

RB   Rebooked

NS   No Show

5. A minimum of two months should be marked off in the appointment book at any one time so that if patients want to book a prime appointment time in advance they may. (Prime times: evenings and Saturday)

6. Develop a waiting list of patients who requested a time that was not available. This list should contain their full name, and work and home numbers, so that they may be called when an appointment time becomes available. A firm appointment time should always be made and then cancelled if an earlier time becomes available.

7. Keep a list of habitual last-minute patient cancellers; then if they have cancelled two times within a predetermined time period, you could notify the patient that if it occurs again they will be charged 50 percent of the service fee.

Streamlining Medical and Esthetic Services

While many practices spend countless dollars on external marketing efforts, internal marketing opportunities offered by the combination of medical and esthetic services are too often ignored.

The following issues should be reviewed and discussed to ensure that the physician and esthetician are working in a productive, complementary manner, and that potential cross-marketing opportunities are maximized.

1. Establish protocols for physician and esthetician coordination of care.

   While the dermatologist or plastic surgeon may initially refer the patient for skin-care treatment as a means of improving overall appearance, or to accentuate a service they have provided, in many cases the physician loses track of the patient once they have begun a regular skin-care program. As a team the physician and esthetician must determine appropriate intervals for physician follow-up based on the patient's individual needs. Should the physician instruct the patient to return in three months, the esthetician will play a part in ensuring that this follow-up takes place. Similarly, the esthetician should be aware of the physician's instructions for prescriptions.

2. Measure "conversion" rates for patients within the practice.

   The only way to tell if your esthetic practice development plans are effective is to measure their impact regularly. One way to monitor this is to audit medical records for "conversion" from the medical practice to skin-care services, and vice versa. For example, take a look at whether skin-care patients have seen a facility physician, and whether medical patients with skin-care problems are under the care of an esthetician. It is easy to see how you can lose control of this advantage by not monitoring results regularly.

3. Determine how to arrange esthetic consultations for medical patients following their physician visit.

   Instead of relying on the patient to call back after receiving a skin-care regimen "prescription" from the physician, arrange for an esthetician to speak with the patient briefly prior to their departure from the office. This will enable you to establish a relationship with the patient, and perhaps phone them back if they do not follow through on their own. Depending on the space available in the facility, you could escort the patient to the esthetic services area. Many practices also utilize telephone consultations if the patient cannot stay for the face-to-face visit.

⅄ Review and Summary ⅄

Developing and adhering to consistent office protocols will take time and training among all staff in the esthetic office setting. Physicians and staff will perhaps need to adjust to the focus on comfort and communication with the patient. The esthetician will perhaps need to strengthen his or her understanding of how the esthetic policies fit into the greater practice picture.

Remember these three cues for your practice administration plan:

Consistency: Maintain a consistent presentation of the practice with patients and other referring entities.

Patient Service: Differentiate the practice from other similar facilities and inform the patient how you best meet their skin-care needs.

Communication: Develop and maintain effective communication pathways both internally and externally regarding patient care needs. As members of the same team, physicians and estheticians must coordinate care to help patients achieve the skin-care goals they desire.

Ask yourself the following questions:

■ How can you use your telephone contacts to make your practice more attractive to prospective patients?

■ Do you know how to track calls to determine how patients learned of your services?

■ Are you successfully using your cancellation list to accommodate patients who need appointments?

■ Have you discussed with new patients the esthetic scheduling protocols?

■ Have you thought of ways to differentiate your practice by offering superior patient services?

Chapter Eight

Business in a Physician's Office

Inga Ellzey

No discussion of esthetic services in the physician's office would be complete without addressing the subject of payment. No matter how well you set up the esthetic practice, how hard you work to bring in patients, and how skilled you are in your craft, none of it means anything unless you can get paid for the services provided.

In this chapter you will learn details and examples of the following:

1. Reimbursement by third-party payers (Insurance)

   ■ When to bill...when not to bill

   ■ Proper **"CPT" coding** (which stands for Current Procedural Terminology that is used to describe and identify medical services and procedures performed by physicians)

   ■ Proper **"ICD-9" coding** (International Classification of Diseases, used to identify diseases that are treated by physicians)

   ■ Documenting the medical necessity of procedures

   ■ Supervision of staff by physician (Medicare's "incident to" provision)

2. Reimbursement directly from patients

   ■ Providing advance notice to patients of non-coverage

   ■ Collecting payment at the time of service (PATOS)

   ■ How to complete a claim form

3. Dispensing of products in conjunction with your esthetic practice

   ■ The dos and don'ts of dispensing

   ■ Overcoming physician concerns about dispensing

   ■ Inventory control
      * Computer tracking of product sales

   ■ Staff concerns

   ■ Handling Supplies

   ■ Stark II legislation

Reimbursement by Third-Party Payers (Insurance)

A myriad of services can be performed by the esthetician in a medical practice. Some of these services are done to improve the health of the patient's skin, while others are performed to enhance appearance and make the patient feel better. The esthetician and the physician must be extremely cautious in determining whether the service(s) provided to the patient are medically necessary or cosmetic in nature. After all, the insurance company uses the physician's number to track the services rendered.

Who makes the determination of medical necessity?

The physician has the ultimate responsibility to determine whether or not a service is medically necessary (e.g., billable to a third-party payer such as an insurance company) or cosmetic in nature (patient has full responsibility for paying for the service).

Are there guidelines/lists available to help the physician determine what is cosmetic and what is not?

No, unfortunately each managed care insurance company and each private commercial insurance carrier establishes their own guidelines for determination of whether a service is medically necessary or not. There is no universal list.

Managed Care Organizations

For managed care organizations with whom the practice has a contractual arrangement, it is imperative that the office manager or insurance personnel investigate and determine which services that are to be performed by the esthetician are or are not be covered. This is especially important with these types of contracts since many of the services that commercial carriers pay for are not reimbursed by managed care organizations. This could mean that the insurance company may only pay for the service if it was done by the physician.

If you have trouble obtaining a list of non-covered services from the managed care organization (they may tell you that there is no such list), three options are available to you:

1. Look back at the last six months worth of EOMBs (Explanation of Medical Benefits) for each carrier with whom your office has a contract. Look at all the documents to see if the codes you are billing (such as 11900/11901, 11200/11201, 10040, 17360, etc.) are paid. Then make a list of which services are paid or denied (and what the reason for the denial is).

2. If you have no historical data to review, follow these instructions:

   a. Fill out a fictitious claim for code 10040, for example. Add a diagnosis (whether for acne, scars, or whatever).

   b. Attach a copy of your medical record documentation, which would support this claim.

      For each code, have two sample claims and two sample progress notes, one showing a medically necessary visit and one which clearly is cosmetic in nature.

   c. Do this for all services you may bill under esthetician services.

d. Contact a supervisor at the managed care organization. Explain that you have been trying to obtain a list of non-covered services. Since your office is trying to establish appropriate billing guidelines, you want to submit ten to twenty "fake" claims for their review. If these were actual claims and the documentation represented actual progress notes, how would their organization reimburse your office, and which claims would not be paid because they are considered medically unnecessary?

e. Establish a deadline for this process. "Mrs. Supervisor, I appreciate you working with our office on this problem. I am forwarding these claims to you today via special courier. May I expect the results by (give exact date; two weeks from the date sent would be acceptable)? I will mark this in my calendar. If I don't hear from you by then, I'll call you."

You need to force these deadlines, or your office will never get this information. Tenacity is the key to getting anything established with managed care organizations. The squeaky wheel gets the oil!

3. Establish protocols in your office for each code used. The protocol basically tells the insurance carrier under which circumstances your office would bill for a service (when it's medically necessary) and under which it would not (cosmetic).

This is somewhat time-consuming and should be developed by the physician. It should be presented to the medical director of the organization (physician to physician). It is by far the most dynamic solution, but also the most time intensive.

Private, Commercial Insurance Carriers

For carriers with whom the office has no contractual arrangements, whether or not the service is covered should be of no concern to you. The only concern is how to complete the form, sometimes referred to as a **superbill**. (Was the service performed medically necessary or cosmetic?).

The patient is responsible for payment at the time the service is rendered. Getting paid back from their insurance is the patient's problem; however, if your office is willing to interact with carriers with whom your office has no contractual arrangement, you should preverify coverage, annual deductibles, and copayments before the service is rendered. While you are on the phone with the carrier, you can ask if they cover the service you want to provide.

Even if your office decides to bill this non-contracted carrier, you should collect thirty-five percent of the entire bill at the time of service...no exceptions! Why? If the carrier denies part of the claim, at least you have some of the payment. Your office will have a difficult time collecting from the patient for services denied by the carrier. Have you ever heard, "If I had known that my insurance was not going to cover this, I would not have had it done!"

What CPT Codes Should Be Used?

In the following section are the CPT codes that are covered by insurance carriers in selected instances and the guidelines that govern those codes. This is meant only as a guide, and the ultimate responsibility lies with the physician to determine whether or not the services you are providing are medically necessary in caring for the patient, in conjunction with the plans with which you have guidelines.

Acne Surgery

Code 10040   Acne Surgery (e.g., marsupialization, opening or removal of multiple milia, comedones, cysts, pustules)

General Guidelines

1. The code can only be used in conjunction with acne diagnoses.

2. This code should be used when removing or incising and draining small acne cysts, comedones, and milia. Commonly these services are provided with a large sterile needle or comedone extractor. Do not use code 10060/10061 for these services. (This will be covered later in this chapter.)

3. The code is not billed in units based on how many lesions are removed. A flat fee is paid no matter how many lesions are opened or removed.

4. The code has 0 global postoperative days.

Injections

Codes *Intralesional Administration*

NOTE: This code is provided as a guideline for physicians; this does not suggest that estheticians can give intralesional injections.

11900 Injection, intralesional, up to and including seven lesions

11901 More than seven lesions

General Guidelines

1. Injections are billed by using a combination of administration codes and "J" codes.

   ("J" codes are found in the HCPCS book. They are not in the CPT book.)

2. For codes 11900/11901, use one code or the other. Do not use both codes on a single patient visit.

   a. If you injected seven lesions or less, you bill only 11900 at one unit.

   b. If you injected more than seven lesions, you bill only 11901 at one unit.

Note: There may be some variation among carriers regarding these codes and their use. Physicians are encouraged to check contracted carriers for billing guidelines.

3. You do not reflect these codes in units. You get a flat fee no matter how many lesions you inject.

Example: Nine cystic acne lesions are injected intralesionally using Triaminicilone 5 mg (intralesional corticosteroid that reduces inflammation). You bill 11901 at one unit and J3301 at one unit.

Note: Always identify the drug you inject and bill this in addition to the 11900/11901 codes. The drug is identified using the "J" codes. "J" codes are discussed in the next section.

4. Codes 11900 & 11901 both have 0 global postoperative days.

"J" Codes—Cost of Drug Codes

General Guidelines

1. "J" codes are special codes that specifically identify drugs. "J" codes are not found in the CPT book. They are listed in the HCPCS book (1996/1997). The codes are considered "Medicare's National Level II Codes."

2. The HCPCS codes are updated annually, as is the CPT book. Physicians are encouraged to purchase a new book at the beginning of each year to stay current on these codes.

   Updates are also provided in the monthly Medicare carrier bulletins.

3. "J" codes are now recognized by many non-Medicare carriers since they are so specific. Physicians should contact any carrier with whom they have a contract and verify whether or not that organization acknowledges HCPCS codes.

4. The "J" codes list generic versions of name brands, when available.

5. The codes specify the basic dosage. Any amount up to and including the dosage is billed as one unit. (i.e., Kenalog is Triamcinolone (TMC) up to 10 mg (J3301). If you gave 1 cc of TMC 5 mg you bill J3301 at one unit.)

Example 1: The physician administers a 5 mg solution of Triamcinolone Acetonide (total 1 cc) intralesionally. The office cannot bill a half-unit on the claim form, so bill one unit of J3301 since it includes any dose up to and including 10 milligrams.

Note: When more than the basic unit dosage is given, bill the code at one unit for each dosage over and above the basic unit dose.

6. "J" Codes are now subject to the Medicare fee schedule.

   a. Effective January 1, 1994, drugs and other biologicals provided by a Medicare nonparticipating or participating physicians will be subject to the Limiting Charge provisions and approved fee schedule.

   b. Fee schedule amounts are based on average wholesale costs as published in the Red Book.

   c. To obtain a Red Book:

Call:	(800) 678-5689 or
Write to:	Red Book Orders
	P.O. Box 10689
	Des Moines, IA 50336

   The book costs approximately $50.

Incision & Drainage

NOTE: This code is provided as a guideline for physicians; it does not suggest that estheticians perform incisions and drainages (I & D's).

Codes 10060 Incision and drainage of abscess (e.g., carbuncle, suppurative hidradenitis, cutaneous or subcutaneous abscess, cyst, furuncle or paronychia); simple or single

10061 ; complicated or multiple

General Guidelines

1. The criteria that make an Incision & Drainage complicated are any one of the following:

    a. The lesion is large.

    b. The lesion requires packing or insertion of a drain.

    c. The procedure is performed in a hospital setting.

    d. The lesion most probably will require redraining during the global postoperative period of ten days.

2. Code all multiples under 10061.

Example: Patient comes to office for Incision & Drainage of a small sebaceous cyst of the eyelid. Patient also has one large abscess of the left malar (cheek area). A drain was inserted.

Note: The physician bills only 10061 at one unit because the definition of 10061 states "multiple."

3. Sac removal may be billed under 11400-11446.

4. All Incision & Drainage codes have ten global postoperative days.

Note: All postoperative time frames indicated in this chapter are based on Medicare's global surgical package since the majority of the United States insurance companies follow the Medicare postoperative time frames. Readers, however, should always verify the postoperative time frames with each managed care contract that has been signed by the physician.

Cryotherapy

NOTE: This code is provided as a guideline for physicians; it does not suggest that estheticians can perform cryotherapy.

Codes 17340 Cryotherapy (CO_2, slush, liquid N_2), for acne
Note: This is a definition revision for 1994.

General Guidelines

1. This code is used only for claims with a diagnosis of acne.

2. This code is not to be used to destroy individual lesions (e.g., keratosis).

3. Many carriers do not pay for code 17340 as they consider it medically unnecessary. Physicians are encouraged to verify coverage with their managed care organizations for coverage guidelines.

4. This code has ten global postoperative days.

Chemical Peel

NOTE: This code is provided as a guideline for physicians, it does not suggest that estheticians can perform chemical peels.

Codes 15788 Chemical peel, facial; epidermal
  15789 Dermal
  15792 Chemical peel, non-facial; epidermal
  15793 Dermal

General Guidelines

1. Any combination of the codes may be used depending on the anatomical location or the depth of the peel.

2. The medical record should clearly indicate the area peeled. Anatomical charts are recommended.

3. The medical record should indicate the strength of the chemical(s) used.

4. The peel process should be adequately documented, including risks, the procedure, and the postoperative instructions given.

5. The record should clearly indicate if the peel was dermal or epidermal.

6. Medicare and many other carriers do allow coverage for chemical peels. Most claims will be pended to determine medical necessity. Claims for chemical peels cannot be preauthorized.

7. These codes have ninety global postoperative days.

Chemical Exfoliation

Codes 17360 Chemical exfoliation for acne (e.g,. acne paste, acid)

General Guidelines

1. This code is used only for claims with a diagnosis of acne.

2. This code is not to be used to destroy individual lesions.

3. Many carriers do not pay for code 17360 as they consider it medically unnecessary. Physicians are encouraged to verify coverage with their managed care organizations for coverage guidelines.

4. Many carriers considered this code a non-covered service. In the case of non-covered services, the patient should be advised in a form signed acknowledging the patient understands their plan does not cover this service, they will be required to pay at the time the service is rendered, and no reimbursement will be forthcoming from their plan.

5. This code has ten global postoperative days.

Electrolysis

Codes 17380 Electrolysis epilation, each hour

General Guidelines

1. This code is billed at one unit for each thirty minutes of epilation.

   Example: You perform one hour of epilation.

2. Time should be clearly documented in the medical record.

3. Medicare and most managed care organizations do not cover this service.

4. No global postoperative days are listed. (This is due to the fact that no insurance carrier will cover this service.)

What ICD-9-CM Codes Should Be Used?

There can be many diagnostic codes associated with these services. Below, the most common diagnoses relative to the five procedures listed above are:

Acne:	
Conglobata	706.1
Cystic	706.1
Decalvans	704.09
Frontalis	706.0
Keloidalis	706.1
Necrotica	706.0
NOS	706.1
Occupational	706.1
Pustular	706.1
Rosacea	695.3
Tropical	706.1
Varioformis	706.0
Vulgaris	706.1
Actinic Keratosis	702.0
Aging skin	701.8
Blackhead(s)	706.1
Comedone(s)	706.1
Cicatrix, skin	709.2
Colloid Milium	709.3
Comedone	706.1
Cyst, skin (epidermal) (epidermoid)	
(inclusion) (epithelial) (retention) (sebaceous)	706.2
Epidermal	706.2
Cholesteatoma	706.2
Sebaceous	706.2
Chloasma	709.00
Skin	709.00
Dilated Pore	701.3
Elastic skin	756.83
Elastosis	
Actinic, solar	692.79
Atrophicans	701.8
Perforans serpiginosa	701.1
Reactive perforating	701.1
Senilis	701.1
Giant Pore	701.3
Hyperpigmentation	709.00
Hypopigmentation	709.00
Macules and papules	709.8
Melasma	709.00

Milia (milium)	706.1
(also Sebaceous cyst)	
Colloid	709.3
Eyelid	373.84
Nodules (cutaneous)	782.2
Skin, NEC	782.2
Papules, fibrous, nose	216.3
Papules	709.8
Perioral Dermatitis	695.3
Pustule	686.9
Rosacea (acne) (keratitis)	695.3
Scar (scarring)	709.2
Atrophic	702.9
Hypertrophic	709.2
Keloid	701.4
Painful	709.2
Sebaceous Cyst	706.2
Sebaceous Gland Disease	706.2
Sun-damaged skin	692.71
Weathered skin	692.79
Wrinkling skin	701.8
Xerosis, skin	706.8

Chart Documentation to Substantiate Medical Necessity

The documentation of services in the patient's medical chart is important for many reasons, this includes substantiation of the services that have been billed (an audit trail) and **medico-legal protection** (insulating yourself and the physician from malpractice suits).

Although there is no magic formula as to what the record should include, physicians (and estheticians who documented in charts) must be aware of the CPT guidelines for E/M (evaluation and management) services. These are clearly stipulated in the front section of the annual CPT coding manual published by the AMA.

There are three components to every E/M service: history, examination, and medical decision making (deciding on what to do with the patient and doing it...like performing acne surgery). These components are referred to as the *key components*. For new patient visits, all three of the key components must be documented.

Sample Chart Note

Patient Name _____ Date _____

History and Physical Examination

	Past Medical History
Chief Complaint	Medications
	Allergies
Physical Examination	Social History
HAIR	
NAILS	Family History
MUCOUS MEMBRANES	
SKIN	
DIAGNOSIS	TREATMENT / LAB

Sample Acne Flow Chart

Name: _____

Date: _____ TX: _____

Skin Type: _____

Comedones: _____

Pustules: _____ Other TXs: _____

Cysts: _____

Milia Cysts: _____

_____ Comments: _____

_____ _____

_____ _____

_____

Other Abnormalities: _____

Medication update: AM _____

PM_____

Alternate _____

Products Dispensed:

_____

_____

_____

_____

_____

Sample Medical History Form
(To be filled out by patient)

Name_____ Date _____

Home Phone_____ Business Phone _____

City_____ State_____ Zip code _____

Date of Birth___ /___ /___   Sex M F Height _____Weight _____

Name of Spouse_____ Closest Relative _____

If you are completing this form for another person, what is your relationship to that person? _____

Referred by Dr. _____

For the following questions, circle yes or no, as applicable. Your answers are for our records only and will be kept in strict confidence. Please note that during your initial visit, you will be asked some questions about your responses to this questionnaire, and there may be additional questions concerning your health.

1. Are you basically in good health?   Yes   No

2. Has there been any change in your general health
   within the past year?   Yes   No

3. Your last physical examination was on_____

4. Are you now under the care of a physician?   Yes   No
   If so, what is the condition being treated?

   _____

   _____

   _____

5. The name and address of your physician is:

   _____

   _____

   _____

6. Have you had any serious illness or operation, or been
   hospitalized in the past five years?   Yes   No

7. Are you taking any medicine(s) including non-prescription
   medicine?   Yes   No
   If so, what medicine(s) are you taking?

   _____

   _____

   _____

8. Do you have or have you had any of the following diseases
   or problems?

   a) Damaged heart valves or artificial heart valves, including
      heart murmur or rheumatic heart disease   Yes   No

    b) Cardiovascular disease (heart trouble, heart attack, angina, coronary insufficiency, coronary occlusion, high blood pressure, arteriosclerosis, stroke)   Yes No

      1. Do you have chest pain upon exertion?   Yes No

      2. Are you ever short of breath after mild exercise or when lying down?   Yes No

      3. Do you have congenital heart defects?   Yes No

      4. Do you have a cardiac pacemaker?   Yes No

    c) Allergy   Yes No

    d) Sinus trouble   Yes No

    e) Asthma or hay fever   Yes No

    f) Fainting spells or seizures   Yes No

    g) Persistent diarrhea or recent weight loss   Yes No

    h) Diabetes   Yes No

    i) Hepatitis, jaundice, or liver disease   Yes No

    j) AIDS or HIV infection   Yes No

    k) Thyroid problems   Yes No

    l) Respiratory problems, emphysema, bronchitis   Yes No

    m) Arthritis or painful swollen joints   Yes No

    n) Stomach ulcer or hyperacidity   Yes No

    o) Kidney trouble   Yes No

    p) Tuberculosis   Yes No

    q) Persistent cough or cough that produces blood   Yes No

    r) Persistent swollen glands   Yes No

    s) Low blood pressure   Yes No

    t) Sexually transmitted disease   Yes No

    u) Epilepsy or other neurological disease   Yes No

    v) Problems with mental health   Yes No

    w) Cancer   Yes No

    x) Problems with the immune system   Yes No

9. Have you ever had abnormal bleeding?   Yes No

   Have you ever required a blood transfusion?   Yes No

10. Do you have any blood disorder such as anemia?   Yes No

11. Have you ever had any treatment for a tumor or growth?   Yes No

12. Are you allergic or have you had a reaction to:

    a) Local anesthetics   Yes No

    b) Penicillin or other antibiotics   Yes No

    c) Sulfa drugs   Yes No

    d) Barbiturates, sedatives, or sleeping pills   Yes No

    e) Aspirin   Yes No

f) Iodine   Yes   No

g) Codeine   Yes   No

h) Other_____

13. Have you had any serious trouble associated with any
    previous dental treatment?   Yes   No

    If so, please explain

14. Do you have any disease, condition, or problem not listed
    above that you think I should know about?   Yes   No

15. Are you wearing contact lenses?   Yes   No

16. Are you wearing removable dental appliances?   Yes   No

17. Are you interested in learning about cosmetic
    services for specific conditions, such as:

    a) Problematic skin care   Yes   No

    b) Sun-damaged skin   Yes   No

    c) Cosmetics   Yes   No

    d) Proper skin care   Yes   No

Women

18. Are you pregnant?   Yes   No

19. Do you have any problems associated with your
    menstrual period?   Yes   No

20. Are you nursing?   Yes   No

21. Are you taking contraceptive pills?   Yes   No

Men

22. Do you have a history of urinary retention or prostate
    enlargement?   Yes   No

    Chief complaint: _____

    _____

    _____

I certify that I have read and understand the above. I acknowledge that my
questions, if any, about the inquiries set forth above have been answered to
my satisfaction. I will not hold Dr. _____, or any other member
of his/her staff responsible for any errors or omissions that I have made in the
completion of this form.

_____

Signature of Patient   Date

For the **established patient** (a patient who has been rendered professional services within the last three years) only *two of the three key* components need to be documented in the medical record; any two of the three in any combination. For the most part, the two most commonly documented key components are the examination and medical decision-making.

An established patient is one where the past history of the patient is already known as well as the medical conditions for which the patient has consulted the physician. Therefore, when the patient returns, in most cases, the patient is examined to determine the status of the condition, and then based on the findings of that examination, a medical decision-making activity is performed. Should the patient continue on the same medications, should one of the medications be increased or decreased, and should any procedures be performed?

The CPT Code 99211 has only the most minimal requirements. A sample of how a chart note might look is provided below:

Sample Documentation

History: Patient returns for acne of the face and back.

Examination: Face shows many new comedones and few cystic lesions. Back much better, with only a few inflamed cysts seen.

Medical Decision Making: Continue on benzoyl peroxide twice a day (BID), acne aid soap. Will do acne surgery and chemical exfoliation today.

How Are Procedures Documented?

The key to properly documenting the procedures depends on what the procedure is and what the CPT states in its definition.

Let's take a look at some of the more common services that would be provided by the esthetician and define the criteria that should be contained in the medical record. Remember, it's not how much you write, but what you write.

Acne Surgery (Code 10040)

Since the definition includes the opening or removal of multiple milia, comedones, cysts, pustules, your documentation needs to identify what was opened or removed and which method was used. It is not necessary to mention how many were treated, but location should be included for medico-legal reasons.

Sample Documentation

Procedure:	Acne Surgery
(DX) Diagnosis:	Acne Vulgaris
Site:	Nasal and malar region
Method:	Comedone extractor
Lesions:	Multiple comedones, milia

A picture is worth a thousand words. It certainly helps to make the record even more valuable if you had a body diagram and noted where the acne surgery was performed.

If a diagram was used, you could simply write "acne surgery with comedone extractor for milia." That would suffice.

Intralesional Injections (Codes 11900/11901)

The definition of these two codes states that it is an "injection"; it mentions the number of lesions (up to seven or more than seven) and then uses the term *lesions*. That's the clue to what is needed to be documented.

Sample Documentation

Procedure:	Intralesional injections TMC 5 mg x cc
DX:	Cystic acne
Site:	Cystic lesions chin
# Lesions:	3
Disp:	RTC (return to clinic) x 2 weeks

Incision and Drainage (code 10060/10061)

The definition of these two codes includes the types of lesions that are included under this code. They are abscess, carbuncle, cysts, furuncle, or paronychia. It also states whether the I & D was simple versus complicated. Finally, it distinguishes between a simple I & D versus a complicated one. (The codes were discussed in detail on page 159.)

Sample Documentation

Procedure:	I & D using #11 BP sterile blade
DX:	Sebaceous cyst
Site:	Left cheek, chin and back
(Anes)Anesthesia:	None
# Lesions:	4
Complicated:	No
Disp.	RTC x 2 weeks

Cryotherapy (Code 17340)

The definition of this code indicates the use of CO_2, LN_2 or a slush procedure limited to the diagnosis of acne.

Sample Documentation

Procedure:	Cryotherapy
DX:	Acne
Site:	Face
Disp:	RTC x 2 weeks

Chemical Exfoliation (Code 17360)

The definition of the code includes "chemical" exfoliation with agents such as acne paste and acid and then states the procedure is limited to the diagnosis of acne.

Sample Documentation

Procedure:	Chemical exfoliation
DX:	Acne vulgaris
Site:	Face
Chemical:	Glycolic Acid 30%
Disp:	RTC x 10 days

Electrolysis will not be discussed because it is never covered by insurance.

Who Has to Sign the Chart Note?

The individual who enters the information must sign or initial the note. (Non-standardized Abbreviations can only be used if there is an abbreviations log available in the office policy manual.) If the documentation is entered by non-physician personnel, the physician of care must sign off on the medical record (sign his/her name under the signature or abbreviation of the non-physician scribe).

Supervision of Non-Physician Personnel by the Provider of Care

Does the physician need to be in the examination room during the time the patient is seen?

No, the physician does NOT need to see the patient personally. (NOTE: This varies by carrier. Careful review of your manged care guidelines is a must to assure compliance.)

Does this individual need any type of special license in order to provide these services for the physician?

No, however, this is a gray area. The esthetician should work within the realm of his or her licensing and not overstep the boundaries.

Medicare's "Incident to" Provision

Medicare has established a specific rule to address ancillary staff performing services on behalf of the physician or provider of care. This rule is referred to as the "**incident to**" provision. It is summarized below.

General Information

Medicare absolutely prohibits a physician billing for services when he or she is *not physically present in the office*. Specifically, Medicare states in Section 2050.2, "Commonly furnished in physicians' offices—Coverage of services 'incident to' the professional services of a physician in private practice is limited to situations in which there is direct physician supervision. This applies to services of auxiliary personnel employed by the physician and working under his or her supervision, such as nurses, non-physician anesthetists, psychologists, technicians, therapists, including physician therapists and other aides. Thus, where a physician employs auxiliary personnel to assist him or her in rendering services to the patients and includes the charges for the services in the physician's own bills, the services of such personnel are considered to be 'incident to' the physician's services. Direct personal supervision in the office setting does not mean that the physician must be present in the same room with the aide. However, the physician must be present in the office suite and immediately available to provide assistance and direction throughout the time the aide is performing the services."

Medicare Section 2050.2 states:

a. Staff can perform services on behalf of physicians.

b. The service can be billed without any modifiers or reductions in fee.

c. To meet the supervision criteria, the physician must be physically in the office or facility, close enough to hear someone calling for help. Being on a separate floor or in a hospital does not meet the definition.

d. Although the physician must be close by, he or she is not required to see the patient.

For non-Medicare patients, there are no state or federal regulations that prohibit a physician from letting his or her staff perform services when the physician is not present in the office. Concern here should be one of liability. What if something went wrong and you were sued—can you imagine the consequences?

Make sure you check any contracts you have with health maintenance organizations (HMOs), physician provider organizations (PPOs), etc. There may be a clause in the contract that requires the physician's presence. Ancillary staff cannot bill for medical services. Different regulations can apply for PAs (physician assistants), nurse practitioners, licensed physical therapists, and other "non-physician" personnel.

Cosmetic Services that Are Medically Unnecessary:

Receiving Payment Directly From the Patient

Physicians and estheticians who provide cosmetic (medically unnecessary) services should always collect for these services at the time of service. That's the beauty of doing non-medical services; it increases cash flow into the practice instead of having to interact with insurance companies which is costly, time-consuming, and requires months of waiting before discounted payment is received.

Physicians who want to develop a cosmetic component in their practices must develop strict financial policies with regard to payment. Because cosmetic services are elective, patients must be told in advance that they are financially responsible. There should be absolutely no exceptions to the payment at the time of service policy for cosmetic services.

Providing Cosmetic Services to Managed Care Patients

If your office provides cosmetic services to patients who are members of a managed care organization, you will need to investigate the rules of your contract. Managed care contracts often place restrictions on physicians who perform services not covered by the plan. Here are some of the things your office will need to obtain answers for:

1. Is there any documentation (a special form) that managed care patients must sign indicating that they understand that the service they are about to receive will not be covered by their plan?

   a. If there is no special form, is a form required at all?

   b. If a form is required, would the Physician Advance Waiver form used for Medicare patients be acceptable?

   This form may be acceptable to the managed care organization. Have them look it over to confirm that the form meets their needs.

   Remember, without proper forms (documentation) you may find you are unable to obtain reimbursement from the contracted carrier or unable to bill the patient.

2. Does your managed care contract have a *balance billing* stipulation? Many contracts do not allow physicians to collect for services at the time of service. The physician must first bill the carrier, get a denial and then balance bill the patient. If the physician has such a contract, it will need to be renegotiated. In renegotiating, advise them that plastic surgeons on their panel are not required to balance bill patients for facelifts or breast implants. Why then should your office have a different requirement when both specialties are dealing with cosmetic (non-covered) services?

   This is a very important issue, since these balance billing stipulations can cause a lot of problems in the office if not corrected before you begin providing cosmetic services.

How Do You Complete a
Claim Form for Cosmetic Services?

The medical practice should not be required to submit any claim forms for services that are of a cosmetic nature. (After all, the plastic surgeon does not have to submit a claim form to Medicare or a managed care organization for facelifts.) It is common, however, for patients to request that claims be submitted just in case the carrier might pay for it.

Managed Care Patients

It is highly recommended that no coded receipts of any kind be provided to managed care patients. You should give them a receipt that shows that they have paid the amount, but nothing that can be used to submit to insurance. Even though there are codes (CPT code A9270 and ICD-9 code V50.9) that are used to designate that a service is cosmetic in nature, some patients repeatedly contact the managed care companies when a claim is not paid, and finally the managed care company acquiesces and pays some really low payment. You collected five times as much since it was cosmetic, but now since the company has "covered the service", your office is obligated to refund the difference to the managed care patient.

Because of this you never want to give patients any kind of coded receipt that can be used for insurance purposes. You should give them only a receipt to show how much they paid you, if so requested. Do not even use a superbill receipt. Buy one of those receipt books that you get at any office supply store or develop a cosmetic receipt, with absolutely no CPT or ICD-9 codes on it.

Medicare Patients

Providing cosmetic services to Medicare patients is much simpler since the law is very clear.

If a physician determines that a service being provided to a Medicare patient is cosmetic or non-covered, then the patient need only to sign the Medicare Physician Advance Waiver form. (This applies to both participating and non-participating physicians.)

You can readily give Medicare patients a receipt or a completed claim form by following these general guidelines:

1. A medically unnecessary service is considered a non-covered procedure under a tertiary medical care system; therefore, it is the responsibility of the patient.

2. When billing an insurance carrier for a cosmetic service, it is recommended that the claim be completed as indicated below. This assures that the claim will be denied.

   a. V50.9 code is used as the diagnosis (this replaces any ICD-9-CM code)

   V50.9 "Elective surgery for purposes other than remedying health states, unspecified."

b. A9270 HCPCS code is used as the procedure code (it replaces any CPT code).

A9270 "Cosmetic Service or Procedure"

Note: It does not matter what service you are providing; you always replace the regular CPT code with A9270 and use the diagnosis of V50.9.

Always collect your charge for the service in advance!

Dispensing Products in Conjunction With Esthetic Services

Dispensing products in conjunction with your esthetic practice can be fun, convenient for the patient, and profitable for the practice. However, before your practice gets involved several issues need to be investigated and you need a clear understanding of how dispensing must be structured in your office in order to be profitable and legal.

The Do's and Don'ts of Dispensing

In this section, a few helpful hints will be offered that assure that dispensing is fun, convenient, and profitable. (The hints are offered in no particular order of importance.)

Do's

Do let your patients know that your office has these products available. Send product lists in monthly billings, develop a quarterly newsletter, have signs and displays in the office. Many physicians add hundreds of thousands of dollars per year in revenue by dispensing products.

Do collect state tax on these items if they are cosmetic and taxable. Your accountant can give you information about how taxes are collected, tracked, and paid in your state.

Do find out about dispensing laws in your state. Each state regulates prescription and may regulate over-the-counter products and cosmetics. One state, for example, limits the mark-ups on products and devices provided by physicians to their patients. (If you cannot add at least one hundred percent markup, it may not be profitable for the practice to get involved with dispensing.)

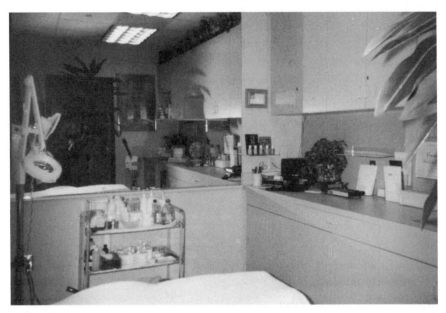

Provide patients with advice on products and an order slip while in the examination room

Do discuss the availability of products with the rest of the staff. Since these products must be purchased, the staff must be aware that they cannot "take" these products home for their personal use or to share with family. Many practices have lost money on in-house dispensing because the profits were eaten up by staff pilfering. The staff should be able to purchase the products at cost but also stipulate that they must order the products through some predetermined mechanism so that the inventory is not depleted.

Do check around for prices before selecting a product line to dispense. Do not get involved with a product unless a fifty percent profit can be made and the product is still competitively priced to the patient for your geographic area.

Do declare confidense in the products you are dispensing:

"Mrs. Avery, I have checked three products on this slip of paper that I want you to purchase. They are products that I have personally investigated and have great confidence in. You may purchase these at the front desk when you check out or you can purchase them from any source you wish."

This phrase accomplishes several important things. It fulfills your obligation of giving the patient a choice. Second, it tells the patient that they need to "purchase" these products.

Dont's

Do not bill for over-the-counter or cosmetic products. Offer patients the options of cash, check, or credit card. If they can't pay now, advise them that they can come back at their convenience to purchase them. Make sure the product recommendations are documented in patients' charts. There should be no exceptions to this rule.

Do not include products that you dispense on your regular encounter form (e.g., Superbill, day ticket, routing slip...whatever your office calls it) unless your office uses these forms only internally. If they are given to the patient as receipts, you should not include these products on them. Develop a separate slip for dispensed products. If you don't, the office will get phone calls from insurance carriers inquiring what type of product it is, what is it used for, etc. in trying to determine if reimbursement to the patient is justified. Cosmetic products are not reimbursable, but your office will spend endless hours answering these requests.

The receipt your office uses should list each dispensed product by name, and there should be something on the receipt that states "not to be used for insurance purposes."

Do not order large quantities in the beginning. Obviously, there may be a financial incentive to purchasing a large quantity since the company from whom you are purchasing will give you a price break if you do so. However, if you are unfamiliar with the product or if the office cannot accurately guess what kind of sales volume to expect once you start dispensing, you should order small quantities to start out.

Nothing reduces profit more than products that sit on the shelf and eventually are thrown out or given away.

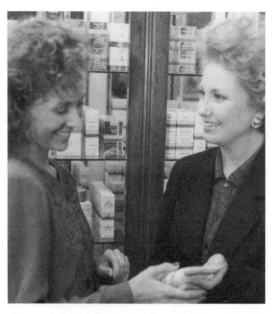

Start out by ordering small quantities of products, until you know what your sales volume will be.

Overcoming the Physician's Concerns About Dispensing

Many physicians are concerned that if they dispense products in their offices, they will strain or even ruin the relationships that they have established with local pharmacists, cosmetic companies, or even other physicians. They do not want to tarnish these relationships in any way since they may rely on these sources for referrals. These concerns are exacerbated in smaller communities where everyone knows everyone. Physicians should be made aware that most patients, even in small towns, purchase skin-care products from large retailers. Such products are not the mainstay of the pharmacy. Obviously, larger chains have more space to dedicate to beauty aides, but pharmacies hardly concern themselves with whether or not your office is competing with them in this regard. Pharmacies make money dispensing prescription drugs.

Inventory Control

Medical practices dispensing over-the-counter products and cosmetics need to incorporate some sort of an inventory control system into the office. If the office has a computer, contacting a local software vendor and finding out whether they have any inventory control systems is the easiest. If not, check with other software companies or stores and try to pick up an inexpensive program that is compatible with your computer hardware.

If the office is not automated and doesn't plan to be, a manual system is mandatory. Items that are used up or considered "consumable"—have an expiration date or lose potency after a period of time—must be carefully tracked so that your office always has enough on hand to meet demand, but not so much that you cannot sell.

With a well-designed and carefully maintained inventory control system, it is easy and almost effortless to track supplies. Without one, it is often virtually impossible to know what is on hand, let alone what should be on hand, how often orders should be placed, and how much should be ordered. (All these factors affect bottom-line profitability.)

It is always best to have a central area where products are stored that is accessible to where they will be given to the patient. (Sometimes, depending on the office design, the storage and dispensing areas may be the same.)

Inventory Log

Grouping products into categories: cleansers, shampoos, moisturizers, exfolliants, sunscreens, and so on, is easy to follow and accessible. When your list of supplies is complete, alphabetize the items in each category. See the example below:

Product Name	Size	Cost	Quantity	On Hand	Order	Sold
XYZ Cleanser	8 oz.	4.90	12	8	6	4

Find out everything about each product, including shipping charges. If you continually run out of a product, you need to place a larger order. Shipping charges can greatly increase the per unit charge when you order three to four times a month. This information is vital to keeping your overhead down.

Keep the inventory list current. Prices can change overnight. Always check the packing slips closely. Using an outdated price list is financial suicide!

Initial Inventory Count

The first time—but only then—you'll have to count everything as the new products arrive. Pay particular attention to expiration dates; if they don't have one, the general rule of thumb is that inventory should turn over every six to eight months. As new products arrive, date-stamp packages before putting them away so you can tell how long they've been on hand. If inventory was already there, you can check the paid invoices to find out how old they are and date the packages accordingly.

During the first couple of months it will be difficult to adjust the inventory, but after awhile you will learn the system and soon have the proper amount of inventory on hand. Keep inventories fairly low in the beginning.

Storage and Handling

Whenever a product is ordered, the terms should be documented on a requisition or purchase order (PO) form. These forms are readily available from most office supply companies or catalogs. The terms listed on the PO should always include unit price, quantity ordered, delivery date, and any special payment arrangements. Also, if the manufacturer or wholesaler offers special pricing or giveaways, be sure to include that information on the PO. Then when the order is received, be sure to check to see if the bill reflects the special offers. It is common for wholesalers to offer special prices or free merchandise for large orders, but then neglect to bill properly based on the special offer.

Another common problem is over-shipment. Any such over-shipments should be promptly returned to the vendor for credit unless you and the supplier can come up with another arrangement. Always make sure that such arrangements are acknowledged in writing. Verbal agreements are not sufficient, especially in large companies where the turnover in personnel is frequent.

Storing and Labeling Products

1. Keep closed packages in dry, preferably air-conditioned and insect-free environments. Moisture, heat, light, and air can damage cosmetic and other health and beauty aids.

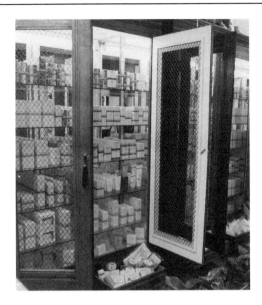

Store closed packages in a dry, preferably air-conditioned, and insect-free environment.

2. If possible, designate a single shelf or part of a shelf for each type of product. (This could coincide with your inventory list.) That way, you lessen the chances of inadvertently reaching for the wrong product. Within each category, separate the products by brands as well as by strength and expiration date, if applicable.

3. Always check to make sure that each product is correctly labeled. If a label should fall off accidentally, be sure to relabel it at once. Unlabeled products should never be dispensed.

   If your office uses a special label, you may want extras on hand in case a label is damaged or comes off.

Handling Supplies... Staff Concerns

Only certain trained individuals should handle (dispense) the products. This is important for a lot of reasons:

1. To assure that the patient receives the correct product.

2. To insure the integrity of the inventory supply system.

3. To assure profit.

How to Track Dispensed Supplies in the Computer

If your office uses a special inventory program, this will be easy to do. However, if your office wants to track the dispensed products within your present medical billing package, you can assign internal codes. These codes can be whatever you want them to be.

Example:	Rejuvenating cleanser	6-oz. tube	11119
	Rejuvenating moisturizer	8-oz. tube	11110

You can make up whatever you want, as long as the codes are used only internally. These codes should not be any kind of CPT or HCPCS (Health Care Financing Administration Common Procedure Coding System) level II codes. They should not appear on any claim form or insurance receipt.

Monthly (or weekly) printouts can tell you how many units you dispensed, at what cost, etc. These printouts can be integrated with your order system and appropriate orders can be placed.

Stark II Legislation and Dispensing

If you dispense any kind of prescription products to Medicare eligible or Medicare beneficiaries, your office must be aware of the **Stark II legislation.** Although over-the-counter dispensing should not be a concern, it is highly recommended that anyone setting up an in-house dispensary contact a health-care attorney to make sure that the structure and all the aspects of the dispensary are legal and do not subject your office to any liability.

A health-care attorney (versus your regular corporate attorney) is recommended for guidance, because the rules are complicated. If you do not know a health-care attorney, you may contact one of the following, whose services can be secured for a reasonable charge:

Alice G. Gosfield and Associates
Attn: Alice Gosfield
2309 Delancey Place
Philadelphia, PA 19103
(215) 735-2384

Geoff Anders
Healthcare Group
Meetinghouse Business Center
140 West Germantown Pike
Suite 200
Plymouth Meeting, PA 19462
(610) 828-3888, Ext. 3316

⭐ Review and Summary ⭐

After reading this chapter the esthetician and physician should be comfortable with the various issues that affect the coding and reimbursement policies of the various insurance companies with which they may have to interact. The importance of the selection of the proper ICD-9 (diagnostic codes) and CPT (procedure codes) cannot be stressed enough.

With increased oversight by Medicare and other insurance companies (especially managed care organizations) through physician audits and utilization screens, office staff and the physicians have tremendous liability in the correct and ethical coding of their services.

Additionally, the importance of proper inventory control tracking should be clearly defined via written policy to assure optimal profitability.

Physicians and estheticians should understand that the policies and rules that govern coding and reimbursement are dynamic. Changes take place almost daily. Readers should therefore be aware that the information in this chapter may be dated. Keeping up with the various changes that govern coding and reimbursement is mandatory.

As yourself the following questions:

- What is a CPT Code?

- What is the difference between an ICD-9 Code and a CPT Code?

- What is a"J" Code?

- What is the procedural difference between a simple I & D and a complicated I & D?

- What are the three documentation components of evaluation and management service?

■ Under what circumstances can ancillary staff perform services on behalf of the physician under Medicare and non-Medicare carriers?

■ Name two ways that you can track in-office dispensing of products.

■ What is the difference between a cosmetic and a drug?

■ Name three "Don'ts" of dispensing products in a medical practice.

■ What is Stark II Legislation, and to what does it refer?

Chapter Nine

How to Promote the Medical Skin-Care Practice

Susan Raef and Ruth G. Sikes

It is important that the esthetician's role in the practice be publicized to patients as early as possible. This chapter is written for the person responsible for marketing the practice; however, it is directed at the physician. The esthetician should be able to assist in compiling the information necessary to put together the marketing plan that will promote the benefits of skin-care treatments.

Are you ready to look at potential patients in a new way? For a moment, take a look inside the mind of a potential patient. Perhaps it's a woman in her early 40s who's concerned about growing lines around her eyes—but dreads the thought of a facelift. Or it may be an aging male executive who wants to keep a youthful appearance for business success.

What probably comes to mind when each of these people thinks of a plastic or dermatologic surgeon? Surgery. But many women and men aren't ready to think about scalpels and sutures.

These individuals are prime candidates for the medical skin-care practice. The physician and esthetician can offer them other alternatives. Perhaps one day they will be candidates for plastic surgery. But in the meantime, you have steady patients—and steady income.

Also think about people with special needs—such as post-chemotherapy patients and burn survivors who need help revitalizing their skin and to feel more confident about their appearance.

And don't forget current patients. Satisfied patients are the best prospects for any business. Patients who have already invested in a facelift, rhinoplasty, or dermatologic treatments are obviously concerned about looking their best.

Now you can help them enhance their new appearance through your esthetician's services. And it's easier to market the new services to current patients—they already know and trust you.

In this chapter you will learn:

■ how to promote a medical skin-care practice

■ how to choose your target markets

■ ways to reach potential new patients

■ how to build a referral network

■ how to form alliances with other health-care professionals

A Practical Marketing Action Plan

There are many potential patients for the medical skin-care practice, but how do you reach them?

1. Identify your target audiences.

   The best way to start is by identifying specific audiences for skin-care services, such as business and professional women, male executives, spa clients, post-chemotherapy and post-radiation patients, burn survivors, and, of course, your existing patient base.

2. Determine your message strategy.

   How will you appeal to these potential patients? Marketers often speak of identifying a **unique selling proposition (USP)**—something that sets one product or service aside from its competition. The USP will become the core of your advertising message.

   Look at the options available to women and men in your community who want professional skin-care services. What are their choices? Day spas? Full service salons?

   What sets you apart from these other options? Medical supervision.

3. Determine your strongest selling points.

In your advertising messages, highlight the advantages of having professional skin-care services medically supervised:

- Before treatment begins, each patient's skin will be evaluated by a physician. (You may want to offer all new patients a skin cancer screening on their first visit.)

- Working as a team, the physician and esthetician will determine a course of skin treatment best suited to the patient's needs.

- The recommended course of treatment will be based on the patient's individual needs—not a pre-packaged series of treatments.

- The physician and esthetician will place special emphasis on making sure each patient understands the recommended treatment procedures.

- The patient's progress will be regularly evaluated by a physician to ensure best results.

- In a medical setting, the patient can be assured that strict sterilization protocols will be followed.

- Patient education materials can help patients understand more about their treatments—glycolic peels, chemical exfoliation, acne surgery, eye treatments, lymphatic drainage, etc.

You should also add selling points specific to your practice—such as convenient location, comfortable office setting, evening and weekend office hours, etc.

A patient satisfaction survey can provide invaluable information for determining your strongest selling point and what other services you should offer.

Reaching your Target Audiences

Now that you have identified your advertising message, how do you reach potential patients? You may want to hire an advertising agency or an experienced freelancer to help you develop an

Sample Patient Survey

XYZ Medical Group
PATIENT SATISFACTION SURVEY

In an effort to advance the quality of our service to you, our patients, XYZ Medical Group is interested in your opinion. Please take a moment to answer the following questions:

1. Would you use evening hours?

   Yes__ No__

2. What hours would you consider using?

   5:00 to 8:00 P.M. _____

   5:30 to 8:30 P.M. _____

   6:30 to 9:30 P.M. _____

   7:00 to 9:00 P.M. _____

   7:30 to 9:30 P.M. _____

3. What days would you like evening hours available? (check as many as you would use)

   Monday_____

   Tuesday_____

   Wednesday_____

   Thursday_____

   Friday_____

4. Would you like office hours on Saturdays?

5. Would you like information on any of the following cosmetic/elective procedures?

   Photoaging skin _____

   Cosmetic Consultation_____

   Acne Skin Care_____

   Collagen Replacement_____

   Liposuction_____

   Laser Resurfacing_____

Please return survey to receptionist. Thank you for your cooperation.

effective promotional strategy. They can also advise you on the best places to advertise in your community, as well as create the marketing materials you'll need—brochures, ads, mailings, etc.

Look for an agency or marketing consultant who already handles some health-related accounts. If you see an ad you particularly like, call the company and ask who handles their advertising.

Many smaller agencies and well-seasoned freelancers do very good work—and don't charge the rates of big-name agencies. Remember, the most important thing is the quality of the advertising—not the name on the door.

It's a good idea to ask for a proposal from several agencies or consultants before making a decision. In your request for proposal (referred to as an "RFP"), outline the skin-care services, as well as the type of promotional support you think you are looking for, such as print advertising, direct-mail, radio ads, speaking engagements, media relations, etc.

Media Relations

Be sure to consider public relations (PR) as well as advertising in your promotional strategy. Often ad agencies or consultants are not set up to do PR. There are, however, many freelance PR professionals you can consider to promote the skin-care practice to the media. PR is very time-consuming, labor-intensive—and greatly dependent on the PR professional's working relationship with local news media. In considering PR consultants, be sure to ask about their local media contacts. The better the working relationship a PR professional has developed with local reporters, the better your chances of getting on the air or in print.

Or you may simply want to ask agencies or consultants to recommend the forms of promotion they think would be most appropriate for the practice. The investment in a good ad agency or consultant will pay for itself many times over.

Print Advertising

Take a look at the publications in your community—city newspapers, business publications, women's newspapers, hospital and community newsletters, etc. Notice whether these publications feature advertisements for skin-care or related services, such as spas, health clubs, etc. Does your Sunday newspaper have a women's section? Or a lifestyle and health section? These are prime avenues for you to promote your skin-care services.

Preparing and placing print ads is best left to the pros. Your ad agency or consultant can develop ads, as well as handle placement in the publications you choose.

Radio Advertising

Think of the radio stations in your market. Which ones are targeted to women ages thirty-five to fifty-four? Or to a professional, upscale audience? To reach these prime prospects, you may want to consider radio advertising. Your ad agency or marketing consultant can help develop and place radio ads. If you're not using an agency, some radio stations will offer help in developing your advertising message—or direct you to appropriate sources. Advertising rates vary from market to market, and by the time of day you want your ad to run. Radio is much less expensive than TV advertising, so don't hesitate to check out the radio ad rates in your market. You may be pleasantly surprised.

Cable TV Advertising

Network TV is probably beyond your advertising budget. But don't overlook local cable TV channels. Before you rule out TV, call your local cable station and find out about their rates and whether they offer any help in producing your commercial.

You may also be able to interest them in doing a feature segment about medically supervised skin care. Let them know they can call you when they have questions about skin-related issues, such as protecting kids from the summer sun.

Local cable stations are always looking for good programming ideas. With a little thought, you can offer them some useful ideas for consumer-oriented programming, which could publicize your skin-care practice at little or no cost to you!

Your Brochure— the "Fulfillment Piece"

A well-written, attractive brochure is a key element of an effective promotional plan. You can ask your ad agency or freelance writers and designers to help create materials that convey your message with style and appeal.

Offer a Brochure in Your Advertisements

A brochure can bolster the effectiveness of your print and radio advertising. In all your advertisements, be sure to offer a free brochure to anyone who wants more information about your skin-care services. Your brochure will be the workhorse that brings new patients to your door.

Who Will Send the Brochures?

Decide well in advance how you will fulfill brochure requests. You may want to have an outside service handle the phone calls, so your office lines won't get tied up, keeping your patients waiting. Ask your hospital's marketing communications department whether they might be able to handle brochure fulfillment for you—or if they can recommend a dependable fulfillment house.

Compile a Prospect Database

Whoever handles your brochure fulfillment, be sure they keep a complete, accurate list of the names and addresses of people who request information about your skin-care services. A mailing list of interested prospects is a valuable asset for any business. These are people to whom you'll want to mail again—so make absolutely certain that a list is maintained in good order. Many excellent computer software packages—such as ACT—make it easy to organize and maintain your database.

Direct Marketing—Your Current Patients Are Your Best Prospects

The patient database of a practicing physician is a gold mine for attracting business for the new skin-care practice. Consider putting together a special mailing to your current patients to tell them about the new skin-care services. You may want to target mailings to specific segments of the patient base—such as women, men, a given age group, or patients with specific diagnoses who would benefit from esthetic treatments, such as acne vulgaris, rosacea, hyperpigmentation, melasma, and photoaged skin. In a plastic surgery practice you will want to target patients who have had facial surgeries such as blepharoplasties, rhytidectomies, and rhinoplasties, and market to their needs for continued skin care to maintain their new look.

The mailing "kit" should include your brochure as well as a cover letter—personalized if possible—to your valued patients. (Personalization is relatively easy with computer software packages you may already have in your office, such as WordPerfect and Microsoft Word. Or you may choose to have a commercial letter shop handle the work for you.)

Make a Special Offer

To show patients you appreciate them—and to encourage them to try the new skin-care services—consider a complimentary fifteen-minute consultation.

Another direct mail idea is to offer skin-care treatments as follow-up care for your postsurgical patients. Once you start thinking about how to interest current patients in the skin-care services, you'll come up with even more ideas for targeted mailings to specific groups.

Follow Up with Your Prospects

Remember the prospect list of people who responded to your advertisements? After several months, mail to them again. Include a cover letter that recognizes they've already expressed interest in your skin-care services.

Offer More Information to Targeted Groups

After your advertising campaign is operating, you may want to think about producing additional brochures on specific subjects—such as "Questions Most Frequently Asked About Glycolic Peels" or "Five Ways to Make Your Face Look Younger Without Surgery". These brochures offer valuable information to key audiences—and promote the skin-care practice and expertise. Be sure your name, address, phone number, and office hours are included on all brochures.

Informational brochures can be very effective in mailings to specific target audiences—such as female patients over age thirty-five. You can also offer them in an advertisement.

Word of Mouth is Still the Best Advertising

Don't forget good, old-fashioned patient referrals. Referrals from satisfied patients are one of the most effective ways to build the medical skin-care practice. Make it easy for your patients to refer their friends, colleagues, and relatives. In your reception area, be sure there's a display of your skin-care services brochure.

Where Did Your New Patients Hear About You?

Keep track of where your new skin-care patients come from. Ask each new patient where he or she heard about you. This will help you gauge the effectiveness of your newspaper and radio advertising. Or perhaps they heard you speak at an association meeting. If it's a referral from a patient—or fellow physician—send a thank-you note to express your appreciation.

Networking: Forming Alliances with Associated Health-Care Providers

Networking is the business buzzword of the '90s. And it works! In your practice, you've no doubt already built successful referral relationships with fellow physicians. Be sure these colleagues and their staff know about your new skin-care services. Take the opportunity to introduce them to your esthetician and offer them samples of your skin-care services brochure.

Build your referral network. Consider who refers patients to you now and what other specialties may have patients who need your skin-care services—such as oncologists or radiologists.

Look beyond medical referrals. You will attract more new patients by extending your skin-care referral network outside the medical community. Consider mailing an introductory letter and several copies of your brochure to non-medical professionals such as image consultants and foreign business consultants—who often advise their clients that their appearance is key to success in business abroad.

Speaking Engagements: Who Is Interested in Your Message?

Where will you speak about your new skin-care services? There are many possibilities. Look in the yellow pages under *associations* or *clubs* to find a list of special interest groups—from professional women to church groups. Another possibility: your state or local medical society auxiliary. Or consider speaking—perhaps in partnership with your esthetician—at health spas in your vicinity. There are also groups of people with special needs—such as those who have undergone chemotherapy, or patients with conditions that alter their appearance, such as alopecia areata or vitiligo.

Preparing for Your First Speaking Engagement

Once you've secured a speaking engagement, you need to target your message to your audience's interests. If you're speaking at a meeting of a women's association, church group, or medical auxiliary, you may want to cover the following topics:

- How to improve skin's texture and appearance.

- How to cleanse and moisturize the skin properly.

- Answering women's questions about professional skin care: What skin rejuvenation or maintenance programs are best for my age group?

- Do I need a peel? What kind? How often?

- How to reduce bags under the eyes without surgery.

- What about liposuction? Who are the best candidates? Are there any good alternatives?

- What are the pros and cons of the most common forms of plastic surgery?

- What alternatives are there to facial surgery?

- Questions to ask your physician before plastic surgery.

- How to apply makeup after having surgery.

- Makeup for the older woman.

For audiences such as post-chemotherapy patients or people with alopecia areata, or vitiligo, you'll need to tailor your remarks to their specific needs and questions, such as:

- How to improve the texture of my skin after radiation or chemotherapy.

- Where to get good wigs from a caring, understanding supplier.

- What alternatives are there to conceal pigmentation abnormalities?

- How to cope with hair loss. What are the alternatives for men and women with pattern baldness?

In preparing your remarks, it's a good idea to start with a simple theme—such as "Ten things you can do to improve your skin's texture and appearance without surgery"—and an outline. If you're an experienced speaker, you may work from bullet points—otherwise, you may want to write your entire speech. Be sure to allow ten to fifteen minutes at the conclusion of your speech for questions from the audience.

Since your subject is so visual, you should include horizontal slides or a personal computer-based graphic presentation to show "before" and "after" pictures to illustrate your point. You can illustrate many points. You may want to ask your ad agency or marketing consultant for help in preparing your remarks or your visual material. Be sure to get a cost estimate so you aren't surprised later.

You may also want to give your audience a simple handout highlighting your major points. Be sure to bring copies of your skin-care brochure. And let the meeting sponsors know well in advance if you'll need any audio-visual material to make your presentation, such as a slide projector, overhead projector, etc.

Prepare, prepare, prepare! Although you don't have to write your entire speech (especially for smaller audiences), don't assume that because you know your subject well, you can get in front of an audience and simply talk. At the very least, you'll want to have a list of "talking points" to help you to follow a logical progression and be sure you cover key topics.

Plan to arrive at your speaking engagement early. Test the microphone, audio-visual equipment, and slides, or have staff check them out. Even the best presentation can be marred by annoying microphone feedback or ill-functioning audio-visual equipment. Be sure you're ready to start at the scheduled time.

Obtaining Media Interviews: How to Interest Magazines and Newspapers

The next time your local newspaper or TV news show runs a story about skin care, wouldn't you like to be quoted as an expert source? It doesn't happen by accident. Successful media relations take a steady, consistent effort.

If you're working with an ad agency or marketing consultant, be sure they know that you're interested in media relations. The first step to working with the media is preparing a "media kit"—a package that introduces you to the local news media, and tells them about your area of expertise. A media kit typically contains:

- A concise, one- or two-page biography (not your entire CV)

- A 5" x 7" black-and-white photo

- One or more news releases

- Reprints of previous newspaper and/or magazine articles where you're quoted or featured

- A copy of your brochure

Reporters are always on deadline. Often they need answers in a hurry. When they're working on a story related to skin care or plastic surgery, they need to know they can count on you to answer a medical question, provide a comment, or be interviewed about a new medical development. You can endear yourself to reporters—and build valuable relationships—by helping to educate reporters and their readers on the medical aspects of skin care. Once you've built these relationships, don't be surprised if you occasionally get a call about a medical story that pops up in the news—such as the "flesh-eating disease" scare. Helping a reporter under a tight deadline is one of the best ways to build positive media relations. And it also keeps your name in front of the public.

Think carefully before making a commitment to be a media spokesperson. You'll need to be prepared to drop everything when the media needs an immediate response, or needs you in the TV studio now.

Media relations is time-consuming work—there are no shortcuts. It pays to have your agency or consultant act as your media liaison.

News Releases

When you send out a news release be sure it's newsworthy and concise. News releases should be double spaced and no more than two pages long. They should contain the name of a contact person and contact telephone number, so the reporter can call for additional information. They also should contain the city and the date of release and contain information about yourself, especially your credentials. Your first paragraph–the "lead"–should spell out the five "W-s" of the news story —who, what, when, where, and why.

News rooms are deluged with news releases from hundreds of organizations every day. To stand out among the mountains of mail and faxes, you have to hook their interest within the first two sentences.

News releases must contain information that will catch the interest of writers as well as readers. For example, it could be about a medical breakthrough or new techniques being introduced into your practice, recently published articles you have written of interest to the public, your election to or nomination for a prestigious office, special public speaking engagements or programs in which you are participating, events in which you are involved that are of local interest, and human interest stories, perhaps about one of your patients (with his/her permission, of course).

If you live in a small town or community, readers might be especially interested in your involvement with community organizations, personnel additions to your office staff, or a new office location. Your consultant can brainstorm with you to pinpoint ideas for magazine or newspaper stories or TV segments.

News releases should be sent before an event is to take place or immediately after. The information provided must be accurate and easy to read.

Familiarize yourself with the kinds of stories that interest the local news media and make a note of the names of the local reporters who cover both medical and health care topics. These are the writers to whom you would send your news release.

Remember—only a small percentage of news releases ever get printed. For the best possible results, make your news releases interesting, timely, and newsworthy.

Sample News Release for Small Hometown Newspaper

ESTHETICIAN'S NAME　　　　　For more information, contact:
(or use your office letterhead)　　Your office manager
Address　　　　　　　　　　　Telephone Number
City, State, Zip
Telephone

DR. SKINCARE, M.D., F.A.C.P., ANNOUNCES NEW ADDITION TO HIS PROFESSIONAL STAFF

CITY, STATE—DATE—Dr. Skincare is pleased to announce the addition of ESTHETICIAN'S NAME to his professional staff. ESTHETICIAN'S NAME brings _____years of extensive experience in the field of skin care. Prior to joining Dr. Skincare, he/she was LIST CREDENTIALS OF ESTHETICIAN.

ESTHETICIAN'S NAME will be a welcome addition to Dr. Skincare's staff and will provide skin-care treatments for special skin problems under the guidance of Dr. Skincare.

Dr. Skincare is a (Diplomate/Member/Board Member/Fellow, etc.) of the NAMES OF ORGANIZATIONS AND ASSOCIATIONS. He/she is affiliated with NAMES OF HOSPITALS. He/she has been in practice in TOWN/CITY at DR'S ADDRESS for ___years. He/she is an active member of COMMUNITY ORGANIZATIONS and (list any awards, offices held, etc.)

Sample News Release for City/Urban Newspaper

ESTHETICIAN'S NAME
(or use your office letterhead)
Address
City, State, Zip
Telephone

For more information contact:
Your office manager
Telephone number

ESTHETICIAN'S NAME to participate in free skin cancer and skin-care consultation as part of a national campaign.

CITY, STATE—DATE—Dr. Skincare and ESTHETICIAN'S NAME, HIS SPECIALTY AND ADDRESS will participate in free skin cancer and skin-care consultations for (any health detection/prevention program) to be held (date) at (location) to coincide with the National Skin Cancer Prevention Day (or any other event) sponsored by Look Good Feel Better.

This (or any other event) is part of a national campaign to encourage early detection and to teach consumers how to take better care of their skin. More than 700,000 people will develop skin cancer this year, and the number is growing by 5 percent per year.

"Your chances of developing skin cancer are one in six," said Dr. Skincare. "Skin cancer can develop in anyone, any age, even young adults. No one is immune from this disease, even though it is usually associated with older people." ESTHETICIAN'S NAME routinely advises his patients on how to properly care for the skin and how to develop good sun protection habits to prevent skin cancer....

For more information on this free consultation program, contact
_____.

Sample Marketing Action Plan

Dr. I.M. Wonderful
Wonderful & Associates
1234 Main Street
Anytown, Anystate 00000

Identifying Target Audiences

Wonderful & Associates has identified business and professional women as the primary target audience for our medical skin-care services, with a special emphasis on existing patients.

Determining Message Strategy—the Unique Selling Proposition

The offices of Wonderful & Associates are conveniently located in the heart of the downtown business district—making it convenient for business and professional women to schedule medical skin-care appointments before work, at the lunch hour, or after work.

Wonderful & Associates recognizes this strategic advantage, and will maximize it by offering office hours to accommodate business and professional women's needs.

Determining the Strongest Selling Points

1. All marketing messages will emphasize the advantages of medically supervised skin-care services—sometimes not available at spas and salons in the area. Before any treatment is given, each patient's skin will be evaluated by a physician.

2. All new patients will receive a complete skin-care screening their first visit.

3. The recommended course of treatment will be based on a patient's individual needs—not on a pre-packaged series of treatments.

4. Patients have the peace of mind of knowing that in a medical setting, strict sterilization protocols will be followed.

How to Reach Target Audiences

Wonderful & Associates will retain XYZ Creative Consultants, Inc. to handle its advertising and media relations.

1. Radio ads aimed at business women will be run during morning and evening commuting times on the local all-news stations. Ads will offer a free brochure for more information on Wonderful & Associates' medical skin-care services and convenient office hours.

2. Space ads will be run in the women's section of the major metropolitan Sunday newspapers, and will feature the brochure offer.

3. All existing women patients ages twenty-five to sixty-four will receive a personalized letter introducing Wonderful & Associates' medical skin-care services, along with the brochure.

4. Wonderful & Associates will introduce their medical skin-care services to physicians and colleagues though a personalized mailing, enclosing a supply of fifty skin-care brochures and an acrylic brochure stand for their offices.

5. Wonderful & Associates will also make an introductory mailing on their medical skin-care services to local image consultants.

Fulfillment of brochure requests will be handled by XYZ Creative Consultants, Inc.

Building Media Relations

XYZ Creative Consultants will prepare a media kit introducing producers and reporters to Dr. Wonderful and his associates, and explaining the advantages of medically supervised skin-care treatment.

Dr. Wonderful will undergo media spokesperson training to prepare him for radio, TV, and print interviews. XYZ Creative Consultants will work on a continuing basis to cultivate media contacts, and promote Dr. Wonderful's availability as an expert source on skin-care stories.

Speaking Engagements

Dr. Wonderful will join the local speakers' bureau, offering his services as a speaker to business and professional women's groups. XYZ Creative Consultants will maintain contacts with these local groups, and cultivate speaking opportunities for Dr. Wonderful.

Sample Press Release

DR. HEALTHY SKINCARE
IS PLEASED TO ANNOUNCE THE ADDITION OF
Cleansing Guru
TO HIS PROFESSIONAL STAFF
CLEANSING BRINGS NINE YEARS OF EXTENSIVE EXPERIENCE
IN THE FIELD OF SKIN CARE. FORMERLY, SHE WAS
PROFESSOR OF AESTHETICS AT SKINCARE SCHOOL,
IN WRINKLE, ELASTICITY
CLEANSING AND HER STAFF WILL CONTINUE TO PROVIDE
SKIN CARE TREATMENTS FOR SPECIAL SKIN PROBLEMS
UNDER THE GUIDANCE OF DR. SKINCARE

(111) 222-3333   444 EAST ACNE CIRCLE
(555) 666-7777   TONER, CA

Sample Brochure/Tri-fold

PANEL 1

WELCOME
To Our Practice

DR. HEALTHY SKINCARE, M.D., F.A.C.P.

Tele. (111) 222-3333   444 East Acne Circle
Fax (111) 666-7777   Toner, California
Tele. (111) 888-9999   1010 Facial Square
Fax (111) 111-1212   Care, California

PANEL 2

Dr. Healthy Skincare, M.D., F.A.C.P.
Diplomate American Board of Dermatology
Diplomate American Board of Internal Medicine
Fellow American College of Physicians
Fellow American Academy of Cosmetic Surgery
Fellow American College of Cryosurgery

Hospital Affiliations
Dermatology Hospital-Skincare University
Cleansing College Hospital

WELCOME
Dr. Skincare and his staff would like to welcome you to the practice. If you have any questions, please don't hesitate to ask. Your questions can be answered by Dr. Skincare, his physician's assistant, his staff of registered nurses, business manager, and estheticians.

PANEL 3

OFFICE HOURS
All patients are welcome to see Dr. Skincare
at either of his offices.

TONER

	Patient Hours Dr. Skincare	Business Staff
Monday	11–6	9–7
Wednesday	11–6	9–7
Friday	8–3	8–6

CARE

	Patient Hours Dr. Skincare	Business Staff
Monday		9–5
Tuesday	8–12	8–5
Wednesday		9–5
Thursday	12–7	9–7
Friday		9–5
Saturday	8–1	8–4

PAYMENT POLICY

Payment is required at the time of the visits. Please feel free to discuss the fees of procedures in advance with our staff.

PANEL 4

INSURANCE INQUIRIES

If your carrier requests additional information or the reimbursement is inadequate, please forward a copy of the correspondence to our office managers to follow up on your behalf. Please remember that this can be time-consuming for our staff, and your patience and cooperation would be most appreciated.

PANEL 5

TEST RESULTS

Certain procedures that are done in the office are sent to outside laboratories for analysis. Patients will be billed separately.

Biopsies
Laboratory: Skincare Laboratory
                 Skincare, USA
Results: Within 7 days of procedure

Bloodwork
Laboratory: Bloodwork Labs
Results: Within 48 hours

Patients will not be called if results are normal. A patient is more than welcome to call our office for the results.

PANEL 6

Dr. Skincare performs all areas of Dermatological Care; including a wide range of surgical procedures.

MEDICAL/SURGICAL	*ELECTIVE*
Acne	Acne Scar Revision
Cysts	Age Spot Removal
Cryosurgery	Collagen
Eczema	Chemical Peels
Electrosurgery	Dermabrasion
Hair Disorders	Fibrel
Infectious Diseases	Hair Transplants
Laser Surgery	Liposuction
Nail Disorders	Nevi
Pediatric Dermatology	Scar Revision
Phototherapy	Skin Care for
Pregnancy Disorders	Problematic Skin
Psoriasis	Tattoo Removal
Skin Cancer	Varicose and
Sexually Transmitted	Spider Veins
Diseases	
Skin Signs of Internal	
Disorders	

No matter what dermatologic problem brought you to this practice; Dr. Skincare and his staff are available to discuss any of your medical concerns.

❧ Review and Summary ❧

In promoting the medical skin-care practice the internal and external ways of marketing have been covered: identifying your target audiences and determining your message strategy. Who do you want to appeal to? This is known as your unique selling proposition, or USP. Determine the strongest selling points of the practice in any advertising message and highlight the advantages of professional skin care. Several points highlight the advantages of the physician-esthetician developing a practice as a team and defining a course of treatment for the patient based on their individual needs, as opposed to a pre-packaged series of treatments.

The emphasis should be on making each patient understand the recommended procedures, including the follow-up given by the esthetician in the home-care treatment. In a medical setting the patient can rely on strict sterilization protocols and that the patient's progress will be monitored by the attending physician.

The final point emphasized is to reach the target audiences. These audiences can be reached by working with an agency or marketing consultant. Print advertising can be effective. Radio or cable TV advertising may be affordable for a single physician or small group practice. The brochure that will be used to promote the practice can certainly go a long way towards bolstering the effectiveness of all other external marketing.

Gathering a database with demographics for the existing patient base and marketing to current patients is always the best prospect. Targeting existing patients and telling them of the new addition to the medical practice can be an effective way to start the new skin-care practice. Offering each patient a complimentary consultation is another great way to introduce the esthetician to the existing patient base. And the best advertising is still word of mouth. Tracking patient referrals and knowing where they come from will help to form alliances with other associated health-care providers and has certainly helped build many referral relationships with fellow physicians. If the esthetician has experience with public speaking, many associations or clubs will find the message very interesting, especially associations of people with special needs. Publishing or obtaining media interviews with beauty editors in newspapers is also a great way to get the word out on the services that the practice offers by educating them on aspects of skin care. Developing these relationships is time-consuming but can go a long way toward promoting the medical skin-care practice.

Ask yourself the following questions:

- Have you pinpointed your target markets: business and professional women, male executives, spa patients, post-chemotherapy and post-radiation patients, and your existing patients?

- Have you determined your unique selling proposition—what makes your skin-care services better than other alternatives available in your community?

- Do you know the media outlets in your area—newspapers, magazines, TV (including cable), and radio? Which ones are best to reach your target audiences?

■ Have you evaluated promotional methods: print advertising, radio ads, direct mail, brochures, speaking engagements, and media relations?

■ Do you know where your referrals come from and how you can expand your patient base?

✤ Appendix ✤

Contents

Sample Medical History Form

(To be filled out by patient)

Name_____ Date _____

Home Phone_____ Business Phone _____

City_____ State_____ Zip code _____

Date of Birth___ /___ /___   Sex M F Height _____Weight _____

Name of Spouse_____ Closest Relative _____

If you are completing this form for another person, what is your relationship
to that person? _____

Referred by Dr. _____

**For the following questions, circle yes or no, as applicable. Your answers
are for our records only and will be kept in strict confidence. Please note
that during your initial visit, you will be asked some questions about your
responses to this questionnaire, and there may be additional questions
concerning your health.**

1. Are you basically in good health?   Yes   No

2. Has there been any change in your general health
    within the past year?   Yes   No

3. Your last physical examination was on_____

4. Are you now under the care of a physician?   Yes   No

    If so, what is the condition being treated?

    _____

    _____

    _____

5. The name and address of your physician is:

    _____

    _____

    _____

6. Have you had any serious illness or operation, or been
    hospitalized in the past five years?   Yes   No

7. Are you taking any medicine(s) including non-prescription
    medicine?   Yes   No

    If so, what medicine(s) are you taking?

    _____

    _____

    _____

8. Do you have or have you had any of the following diseases
    or problems?

    a) Damaged heart valves or artificial heart valves, including
        heart murmur or rheumatic heart disease   Yes   No

b) Cardiovascular disease (heart trouble, heart attack, angina, coronary insufficiency, coronary occlusion, high blood pressure, arteriosclerosis, stroke)	Yes	No
1. Do you have chest pain upon exertion?	Yes	No
2. Are you ever short of breath after mild exercise or when lying down?	Yes	No
3. Do you have congenital heart defects?	Yes	No
4. Do you have a cardiac pacemaker?	Yes	No
c) Allergy	Yes	No
d) Sinus trouble	Yes	No
e) Asthma or hay fever	Yes	No
f) Fainting spells or seizures	Yes	No
g) Persistent diarrhea or recent weight loss	Yes	No
h) Diabetes	Yes	No
i) Hepatitis, jaundice, or liver disease	Yes	No
j) AIDS or HIV infection	Yes	No
k) Thyroid problems	Yes	No
l) Respiratory problems, emphysema, bronchitis	Yes	No
m) Arthritis or painful swollen joints	Yes	No
n) Stomach ulcer or hyperacidity	Yes	No
o) Kidney trouble	Yes	No
p) Tuberculosis	Yes	No
q) Persistent cough or cough that produces blood	Yes	No
r) Persistent swollen glands	Yes	No
s) Low blood pressure	Yes	No
t) Sexually transmitted disease	Yes	No
u) Epilepsy or other neurological disease	Yes	No
v) Problems with mental health	Yes	No
w) Cancer	Yes	No
x) Problems with the immune system	Yes	No
9. Have you ever had abnormal bleeding?	Yes	No
Have you ever required a blood transfusion?	Yes	No
10. Do you have any blood disorder such as anemia?	Yes	No
11. Have you ever had any treatment for a tumor or growth?	Yes	No
12. Are you allergic or have you had a reaction to:		
a) Local anesthetics	Yes	No
b) Penicillin or other antibiotics	Yes	No
c) Sulfa drugs	Yes	No
d) Barbiturates, sedatives, or sleeping pills	Yes	No
e) Aspirin	Yes	No

f) Iodine	Yes	No
g) Codeine	Yes	No
h) Other_____		

13. Have you had any serious trouble associated with any previous dental treatment?   Yes No

   If so, please explain

14. Do you have any disease, condition, or problem not listed above that you think I should know about?   Yes No

15. Are you wearing contact lenses?   Yes No

16. Are you wearing removable dental appliances?   Yes No

17. Are you interested in learning about cosmetic services for specific conditions, such as:

   a) Problematic skin care   Yes No

   b) Sun-damaged skin   Yes No

   c) Cosmetics   Yes No

   d) Proper skin care   Yes No

Women

18. Are you pregnant?   Yes No

19. Do you have any problems associated with your menstrual period?   Yes No

20. Are you nursing?   Yes No

21. Are you taking contraceptive pills?   Yes No

Men

22. Do you have a history of urinary retention or prostate enlargement?   Yes No

   Chief complaint: _____

   _____

   _____

I certify that I have read and understand the above. I acknowledge that my questions, if any, about the inquiries set forth above have been answered to my satisfaction. I will not hold Dr. _____, or any other member of his/her staff responsible for any errors or omissions that I have made in the completion of this form.

_____

Signature of Patient   Date

Sample Acne Flow Chart

Name: _____

Date: _____	TX: _____
Skin Type: _____	
Comedones: _____	
Pustules: _____	Other TXs: _____
Cysts: _____	
Milia Cysts: _____	
_____	Comments: _____
_____	_____
_____	_____
_____	

Other Abnormalities: _____

Medication update: AM _____

PM _____

Alternate _____

Products Dispensed:

_____

_____

_____

_____

_____

Sample Chart Note

Patient Name _____ Date _____

History and Physical Examination

Chief Complaint	**Past Medical History** _____ _____ _____ _____ _____ **Medications** _____ _____ _____ _____ **Allergies** _____ _____

Physical Examination	Social History
HAIR	
NAILS	Family History
MUCOUS MEMBRANES	
SKIN	

	TREATMENT	LAB
DIAGNOSIS		

Sample Daily Close Form

Accounting date: _____

Prepared by (initial after your portion is complete): _____

Encounter forms from _____ through _____

Reception Services

1. Over-the-counter cash $ _____

2. Over-the-counter checks $ _____

3. VISA/Mastercard/Discover $ _____

4. Total: Lines 1 + 2 + 3 $ _____

5. Report total (on deposit slip report) $ _____

6. Over/Under (Lines 4 and 5) $ _____

When lines 4 and 5 balance, the day is balanced.

Plus Any Additional Payments (itemize)

_____ $ _____

_____ $ _____

_____ $ _____

_____ $ _____

_____ $ _____

Total To Deposit $ _____

Sample Referral Questionnaire

How Did You Learn About Skin Care Associates?

Please circle all statements that apply:

1. My friend, _____ told me about _____
2. My doctor, _____ told me about _____
3. Your location is convenient to my home or office.
4. I noticed your yellow pages ad.
5. I noticed your newspaper ad in_____
6. I heard your radio ad on station _____
7. I heard _____ speak at the educational seminar on _____
8. I read your newsletter.
9. Other _____

Sample Telephone Tracking Form

Date/Time Taken: _____

Patient Name: _____

Mailing Address: _____

Phone Numbers: Home (   ) _____

                     Work (   ) _____

Initial Interest: _____

_____

Referred By: _____

Information Sent: _____

Prices Quoted: _____

Date of Visit: _____

Taken By: _____

Sample Procedure Consent Form for Micropigmentation

Name _____Address _____

City _____ State _____ Zip _____

Phone Home (   ) _____ Work (   ) _____

Referred by _____ Procedure_____

Do you take Zovirax?	No	Yes
Do you wear contact lenses?	No	Yes
Do you have any kind of heart trouble?	No	Yes
Are you a diabetic?	No	Yes
Are you taking recreational drugs?	No	Yes
Are you able to take Benadryl?	No	Yes
Are you allergic to novocaine?	No	Yes
Do you get fever blisters/cold sores?	No	Yes
Have you ever tested positive for HIV?	No	Yes
Are you presently taking any medication?	No	Yes

List: _____

Fees discussed _____ Deposit _____ Balance _____
I fully understand that a consultation fee of $50.00 will be deducted from my deposit in the event of cancellation of said procedure. The entire staff is dedicated to client satisfaction. We employ a no-refund policy, and I am aware of this. x _____ Date _____

I absolutely understand that this procedure is a process and subsequent visits are necessary in order to achieve desired results. Subsequent visits are subject to $100/$300 charge depending upon the amount of work needed. It is understood that I have received a patch test prior to application, which releases _____ and assistants from any liability related to any allergic or other reaction to applied pigments.(Pigment contents: iron oxide, alcohol, distilled water, glycerine) I acknowledge that no guarantees have been made to me concerning the results of this procedure. For the purpose of documentation, I also consent to the taking of before-and-after photographs of said procedure, which may or may not be used by _____. I have read the above and had explained to me and fully understand this consent and procedure form: That the explanations therein referred to were made and I accept full responsibility for these or any other complications that may arise from results during or following the cosmetic procedure(s) which is to be performed at my request according to this consent and procedure form. x _____ Date _____

_____
Patient Signature

_____
Physician Signature

_____
Witness Signature

Sample Procedure Consent Form, check with your legal counsel for one which specifically fits your needs.

Sample Consent Form

I hereby consent to and authorize Dr._____and/or his assistants to perform the procedure of _____upon myself.

I fully understand the necessity and/or elective reasoning of this procedure, which has been explained to me by Dr._____and/or his assistants.

As with any procedure, I also understand that there are certain risks involved. These include the possibility of further treatment of the treated sites, hypertrophic and/or keloid scarring, and hyper- or hypopigmentation of the skin.

As far as my treatment course, I understand that there is a chance of swelling, bruising, and/or some mild and/or moderate discomfort which are all normal occurrences of this procedure.

I agree to follow to the best of my ability all postoperative instruction given to me by Dr._____and/or his assistant. I understand that instruction and/or medication involved are for the best healing and cosmesis of the areas treated.

I have also, to the best of my knowledge, given an accurate account of my past medical history, including all known allergies, to Dr._____ and/or his assistant and fully understand the information above.

Date_____

Patient's Signature _____

Physician's Signature _____

Witness _____

Sample Consent Form, check with your legal counsel for one which specifically fits your needs.

SAMPLE NON-COMPETITION AGREEMENT

FOR VALUE RECEIVED and other good consideration, the undersigned

jointly and severally covenant and agree not to compete with the business of

located at

("Company") and its lawful successors and assigns, pursuant to the terms hereof.

The term "not compete" as used herein shall mean that the undersigned shall not directly or indirectly engage in a business or other activity generally described as:

notwithstanding whether said participation be as an owner, officer, director, employee, agent, consultant, partner or stockholder (except as a passive stockholder in a publicly owned company).

This covenant not to compete shall extend only for a radius of   miles from the present location of the Company at   , and shall remain in full force and effect for   years from date hereof whereupon it shall terminate.

In the event of any breach, the Company shall be entitled to full injunctive relief without need to post bond, which rights shall be cumulative with and not necessarily successive or exclusive of any other legal rights.

This Agreement shall be binding upon and inure to the benefit of the parties, their successors, assigns and personal representatives.

Upon breach the undersigned shall be responsible for all reasonable attorneys fees and costs incurred in the enforcement of this agreement.

Special provisions:

Signed under seal this   day of   , 19   .

Signed in the presence of:

_____ _____

_____ _____

Acknowledged by (Company)

_____

Sample Non-competition Agreement, check with your legal counsel for one which specifically fits your needs.

SAMPLE CONFIDENTIALITY AGREEMENT

AGREEMENT by and between

(Company) and   , (Undersigned),

Whereas, the Company agrees to allow the Undersigned access to certain confidential information, trade secrets, or proprietary information relating to the affairs of the Company only for purposes of:

, and

Whereas, the Undersigned and its agents, attorneys, accountants or advisors may review, examine, inspect, have access to or obtain such information only for the purposes described above, and to otherwise hold such disclosed information confidential pursuant to the terms of this agreement

BE IT ACKNOWLEDGED, that the Company has or shall furnish to the Undersigned certain confidential information, described on the attached list, and Company may further allow the Undersigned the right to inspect the business of the Company and/or interview suppliers, customers, employees or representatives of the Company, only on the following conditions:

1.   The Undersigned agrees to hold all disclosed confidential or proprietary information or trade secrets ("information") in trust and confidence and agrees that it shall be used only for the contemplated purpose, and shall not be used for any other purpose nor disclosed to any third party without written consent of Company.

2.   No copies or abstracts will be made or retained of any written information supplied. Upon demand by the Company, all information, including written notes, photographs, or memoranda shall be returned to the Company.

3.   The disclosed information shall not be disclosed to any employee, consultant or third party unless said party agrees to execute and be bound by the terms of this agreement.

4.   It is understood that the Undersigned shall have no obligation to hold confidential with respect to any information known by the Undersigned or generally known within the industry prior to date of this agreement, or that shall become common knowledge within the industry thereafter as said information shall not be deemed protected under this agreement.

5.   The Undersigned acknowledges the information disclosed herein constitutes proprietary and trade secrets and in the event of unlawful use or wrongful disclosure, the Company shall be entitled to injunctive relief as a cumulative and not necessarily successive remedy without need to post bond.

6.   This agreement shall be binding upon and inure to the benefit of the parties, their successors, assigns and personal representatives.

Special provisions:

Signed under seal this   day of   , 19   .

Signed in the presence of:

_____   _____

_____   _____

Sample Confidentiality Agreement, check with your legal counsel for one which specifically fits your needs.

Sample Job Description

Position: Esthetician

Summary: Responsible for performing skin-care services for patients under the supervision of a physician. Assisting in patient care through communication with office staff and the physician.

Responsibilities:

1. Coordinates patient care with the physician, including but not limited to the use of oral and topical medications, pre- and postoperative care, and various patient compliance concerns.

2. Provides new patients with complimentary consultations regarding skin-care services.

3. Serves as a liaison with the patient coordinator during the pre- and post-operative phase of patient treatment to ensure understanding of the outcome.

4. Maintains treatment rooms and work stations in compliance with OSHA standards.

5. Seeks advice of physician on treatment protocols and advises physician of patient noncompliance.

6. Maintains and insures current patient records detailing treatment procedures, products, medications, and educational information.

7. Takes care of equipment for proper operation, including cleaning, as suggested by manufacturer.

8. Overviews and updates office personnel telephone procedure on handling scheduling, confirming appointments, wait listing, cancellation protocols, and patient tracking.

9. Participates and attends in-service programs and staff meetings.

10. Assists with orientation and training of new office personnel, including but not limited to product education, sales procedures, skin-care services, and any other related protocols.

11. Coordinates any correspondence/brochures to patients regarding their skin-care treatments, product usage, and home-care instructions.

12. Tracks outside referral sources and sends thank-you letters and/or post-consultation letters if referred by another physician.

13. Maintains inventory system for professional and retail products and tracking of sales tax.

14. Orders and stocks medical supplies and products as needed for maintaining treatment room and retail shelves.

Sample Cover Letter to Physician

Dear Dr.:

I'd like to take this opportunity to introduce myself to you. I am a licensed esthetician in the State of New York, and I am presently working in a full-service salon, which offers hair, nail and skin-care services.

As an esthetician I perform a variety of skin-care services that help to enhance a client's skin by exfoliation of dead skin cells, cleansing and extraction of comedones, and hydration of the skin. I also have the ability to assist facial-surgery clients in returning to their normal routines by the application of camouflage cosmetics, which cover bruising and redness.

I have gained much experience over the last three years working in a salon; however, I feel that I can best utilize my talents in a medical setting. If you have not already thought about setting up esthetic skin-care services in your practice, I would very much like the opportunity to meet with you and discuss the benefits for you and your patients.

I will call you in two weeks, after you have had a chance to review my resumé, and see when you would like to meet with me. Thank you in advance for your consideration.

Sincerely,

Your name, typed

Enclosure—Resume

Directory of
Professional Associations

Aesthetics International Association
3939 East Highway 80, Suite 408   (214) 526-0752
Mesquite, TX 75150   Fax   (214) 526-2925

American Academy of Cosmetic Surgery   (312) 527-6713
401 N. Michigan Avenue   Fax   (312) 644-1815
Chicago, IL 60611-4267

American Academy of Dermatology   (847) 330-0230
930 N. Meacham Road   (847) 330-0050
P.O. Box 4014
Schaumburg, IL 60168-4014

American Academy of Facial Plastic and
Reconstructive Surgery   (202) 842-4500
1110 Vermont Ave, NW, Suite 220   Fax   (202) 371-1514
Washington, DC 20005-3522

American Aesthetician's Education Association, Inc.
AAEA Headquarters   (214) 394-1740
P.O. Box 117896   Fax   (214) 492-9630
Carrollton, TX 75011-7896

American Beauty Association   (312) 245-1595
401 North Michigan Avenue   Fax   (312) 245-1080
Chicago, IL 60611

American Cleft Palate-Cranofacial Association
1218 Grandview Avenue   (412) 481-1376
Pittsburgh, PA 15211   Fax   (412) 481-0847

American Electrology Association   (203) 374-6667
106 Oak Ridge Road   Fax   (203) 372-7134
Trumbull, CT 06611

American Nurses Association   (202)554-4444
P.O. Box 2244   (800) 637-0323
Waldorf, MD 20604-2244

American Skin Association   (212) 753-8260
150 East 58th Street   Fax   (212) 688-6547
New York, NY 10155-0002

American Society For Aesthetic   (847) 228-9274
Plastic Surgery, Inc.   Fax   (847) 228-9905
444 East Algonquin Road
Suite 110
Arlington Heights, IL 60005

American Society For Dermatologic Surgery, Inc.   (504) 483-6957
Nadine Tosk–Media Contact   Fax   (504) 483-6958
2730 Bell St.
New Orleans, LA 70119

American Society of Esthetic Medicine   (602) 368-0108
7007 E. Gold Dust Ave., Bldg. 6, Suite 2022
Scottsdale, AZ 85253

American Society of Plastic and
Reconstructive Surgeons   (847) 228-9900
444 East Algonquin Road   Fax   (847) 228-9131
Arlington Heights, IL 60005

American Society of Plastic and Reconstructive
Surgical Nurses, Inc.   (609) 589-6247
North Woodbury Road   Fax   (609) 589-7463
Box 56
Pitman, NJ 08071

CIDESCO/U.S.A. Representative
National Cosmetology Assoc.   (314) 534-7980
3510 Olive Street   Fax   (314) 534-8618
St. Louis, MO 63103

Cosmetic, Toiletry, Fragrance Assoc.   (202) 331-1770
1101 17th Street N.W., Suite 300   Fax   (202) 331-1969
Washington, DC 20036-4702

Dermatology Nurses Association   (609) 256-2300
North Woodbury Road   Fax   (609) 589-7463
Box 56
Pitman, NJ 08071

Esthetics Manufacturers and Distributors Alliance
401 North Michigan Avenue   (312) 245-1595
Chicago, IL 60611   Fax   (312) 245-1080

Foundation For Ichthyosis & Related Skin Types
P.O. Box 20921   (800) 545-3286
Raleigh, NC 27619   (919) 782-5728
                                 Fax   (919) 781-0679

International Guild of Professional		(910) 841-6631
Electrologists, Inc.	Fax	(910) 841-5187
202 Boulevard Street, Suite B		
High Point, NC 2726		

Lupus Foundation of America, Inc.   (301) 670-9292
4 Research Place, Suite 180   (800) 558-0121
Rockville, MD 20850-3226

National Alopecia Areata Foundation   (415) 456-4644
710 C Street, Suite 11   Fax   (415) 456-4274
San Rafael, CA 94901

National Cosmetology Association   (314) 534-7980
3510 Olive Street   Fax   (314) 534-8618
St.Louis, MO 63103

National Eczema Association   (503) 228-4430
1221 S. W. Yamhill, Suite 303
Portland, OR 97205

National Psoriasis Foundation
6600 S.W. 92nd Avenue, Suite 300   (503) 244-7404
Portland, OR 97223   Fax   (503) 245-0626

National Rosacea Society   (847) 382-7404
800 South Northwest Highway, Suite 200   Fax   (847) 382-5567
Barrington, IL 60010

National Tuberous Sclerosis Association   (800) 225-NTSA
8181 Professional Place, Suite 110   (301) 459-9888
Landover, MD 20785   Fax   (301) 459-0394

National Vitiligo Foundation, Inc.   (903) 531-0074
P. O. Box 6337
Tyler, TX 75711
Or
100 Independence Pl., Suite 200
Tyler, TX 75703

Nevoid Basal Cell Carcinoma Syndrome   (800) 815-4447
162 Clover Hill St.   (508) 485-4873
Marlborough, MA 01752   Fax   (508) 481-4072

North American Society of Phlebology   (708) 330-9830
930 North Meacham Road   Fax   (708) 330-0050
Schaumburg, IL 60173

Occupational Safety & Health Administration   (202) 219-8151
U.S. Department of Labor
Washington, DC 20210

Scleroderma Federation
Peabody Office Building   (508) 535-6600
One Newbury Street   Fax   (508) 535-6696
Peabody, MA 01960

Society of Clinical & Medical Electrologists, Inc.
132 Great Road, Suite 200   (508) 461-0313
Stow, MA 01775   Fax   (508) 897-5442

Society of Permanent Cosmetics   (707) 586-2982
655 Enterprise Drive, Suite 200
Rohnert, CA 94928

Society of Plastic Surgical Skin Care Specialists
C/O The Aesthetic Society   (310) 595-4275
3922 Atlantic Avenue   Fax   (310) 427-2234
Long Beach, CA 90807

The Phoenix Society For Burn Survivors, Inc.
11 Rust Hill Road   (800) 888-Burn
Levittown, PA 19056   Fax   (215) 946-4788

The Skin Cancer Society   (212) 725-5176
245 Fifth Avenue, Suite 2402   Fax   (212) 725-5751
New York, NY 10016

United Scleroderma Foundation, Inc.   (800) 722-HOPE
P. O. Box 399   (408) 728-2202
Watsonville, CA 95077-0399

Directory of Services

Inga C. Ellzey, MPA, RRA
Inga Ellzey Practice Group, Inc.
1398 Semoran Boulevard
Suite 102
Casselberry, FL 32707
(407) 678-4609 Fax (407) 678-5751

The Inga Ellzey Practice Group provides support in the following areas:

- ICD-9,CPT and HCPCS Coding
- Interaction with third-party payors (HMOs, PPOs, IPAs, etc.)
- Medicare compliance
- Medical record documentation
- Billing and collections procedures and processes
- Insurance claims processing
- Personnel related issues
- Automation need determination and selection
- Product development (administrative/clinical)
- A bimonthly newsletter, i.e., with a present subscribership of 2,000
- A list of specialty products developed to meet the needs of the practicing dermatologist
- A national billing service for dermatologists

M. Susan Raef
WordPower Communications, Inc.
30 E. Huron Street
Suite 2809
Chicago, IL 60611
(312) 951-6110 Fax (312) 951-0450

Susan Raef is president of WordPower Communications, Inc., a Chicago-based marketing communications firm she founded in 1994. She is the former director of the American Medical Association's Department of Communications Services. Ms. Raef is in demand as a health-care marketing strategist and writer, with an emphasis in direct marketing.

Ruth Sikes
Sikes & Associates
2615 West Birchwood
Chicago, IL 60645
(773) 274-0043 Fax (773) 274-4047

Ruth Sikes has been a communications professional for more than twenty years. Until 1993, she was with the American Academy of Dermatology as Assistant and then Acting Director of Communications. Today, Ms. Sikes is a consultant and writer, creating public relations campaigns, print and audiovisual materials, and consumer articles on health and skin care.

Susanne S. Warfield
Paramedical Consultants, Inc.
15 North Broad Street
Ridgewood, NJ 07450-3801
(201) 670-4100 Fax (201) 670-4265

Paramedical Consultants, Inc. provides on-site consultation to the physician who wants to establish or evaluate the use of estheticians in their practice. The development of unique products for your practice as well as guidance in setting up in-office dispensing. Our placement service of estheticians assist in staff recruitment and containment.

Sarah Wiskerchen
Karen Zupko & Associates
625 North Michigan Avenue
Suite 702
Chicago, IL 60611-3110
(312) 642-5616 Fax (312) 642-5571

Sarah Wiskerchen of Karen Zupko & Associates works extensively with dermatologists and plastic surgeons nationwide, helping them to develop their practices.

Directory of Professional Publications

COSMETIC DERMATOLOGY   (800) 783-4903
105 Raider Blvd.   Fax   (908) 874-5041
Bell Mead, NJ 08502

DERMASCOPE
The Encyclopedia of Aesthetics   (214) 682-9510
3939 E. Highway 80, Suite 408   Fax   (214) 686-5901
Mesquite, TX 75150

DERMATOLOGY NURSING   (609) 256-2300
East Holly Avenue   Fax   (609) 589-7463
Box 56
Pitman, NJ 08071-0056

LES NOUVELLES ESTHETIQUES   (800) 471-0229
306 Alcazar Avenue, Suite 204   (305) 443-2322
Coral Gables, FL 33134   Fax   (305) 443-1664

PCI JOURNAL OF PROGRESSIVE CLINICAL INSIGHTS
15 North Broad Street   (201) 670-4100
Ridgewood, NJ 07450   Fax   (201) 670-4265

PLASTIC SURGICAL NURSING   (609) 256-2340
East Holly Avenue   Fax   (609) 589-7463
Box 56
Pitman, NJ 08071-0056

SKIN INC.   (708) 653-2155
362 South Schmale Road   Fax   (708) 653-2192
Carol Stream, IL 60188-2787

❋ Index ❋

F

Fibroblasts, 27
Follow-Up letter, 87-88

G

Garamycin gauze, 30
Gelling agents, 23
Glycolic alpha-hydroxy acid, 31

H

Hair loss, 30
Hydrating masks, 23-25. (See also Masks)
Hypertrophic scars, 30
Humectants, 24

I

ICD-9 coding, 151, 162-63
"Incident to" provision, Medicare, 154, 173-74
Incision & Drainage CPT code, 159
Independent contractor, 11-12, 103-6, 122
Informed consent, 124-27
Injections, CPT code, 157
International Classification of Diseases. (See ICD-9 coding)
Interview, 77-88
    cold call, 78-80
    gatekeepers, 80-83
    getting the, 77-78
    phone, 83
    preparation for, 84
Intralesional Administration codes, 157
IRS employment status, determining, 103-4
Itching, 31

J

"J" CPT code, 158
Jessner Peels, 31
Job description, formulating, 57
Job description, sample, 222

K

Kaolin, 22
Key components, 163

L

Lactic alpha-hydroxy acid, 31
Letter, cover, 69-73
Letter, follow-up, 87-88
Leukopenia, 29
Liability insurance, 102, 119-130
    independent contractors, 122
    informed consent, 124-27
    professional advice, 120-22
Lymph, 16
Lymphatic drainage massage, 16-19
Lymphobiology, 19-21
    benefits, 19-20
    double blind study, 20
    efficiency, 20
    postoperative considerations, 21
    procedure, 20-21
    safety, 20

M

Macrophages, 27
Managed Care organizations, 153-54, 174-76. (See also Reimbursement)
Manual Lymph Drainage, 17-19
    basic hand movements, 17
    contraindications, 18-19
    developers, 17
    indications, 18
    length of treatment, 17
Marketing. (See Promotion)
Marketing Action Plan, sample, 201-3
Masks, 21-25
    acneic skin, 22-23
    definition, 21-22
    hydrating, 23-25
    purpose, 22
Medical History Form, sample, 166-68, 210-12
Medical insurance, 99-101. (See also Employment Agreement)
Medical procedures
    preparing the skin, 5-7
Medicare
    cosmetic services, 176-77
    "Incident to" provision, 154, 173-74
    Stark II legislation, 184-85
Medico-legal protection, 163

Style. Savvy. Solutions.

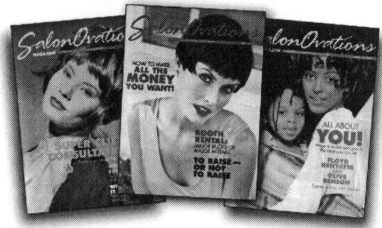

every month.

SalonOvations

SalonOvations is a professional and personal magazine designed with you in mind. Each issue delivers great features on personal growth and on-target stories about the beauty business. Get helpful hints from industry pros on starting your own salon business and how to satisfy your clients. Plus, you'll get pages of colorful photos of the latest trends in haircutting, styling and coloring.

All this at a great price of $22 15 issues for only $19.95 a year! **3 FREE issues** - Save over 40%

(price subject to change)